THE ONE HABIT DIFFERENCE:

HOW ADDING ONE HABIT CAN LEAD TO A LIFETIME OF GOOD HEALTH

TABLE OF CONTENTS

Optimal health is merely a series of habits implemented over the course of a lifetime. Our bodies will naturally adapt to our environment for better or worse. Humans are resilient creatures - we can endure a lot without realizing it. The compounding effects of poor health are all around us. Lifestyle diseases - including heart disease, cancer, and chronic lower respiratory disease, are on the list of the top eight causes of death today. Contrast this with one hundred years ago, when communicable diseases were much more prevalent, and the top three causes of death were pneumonia/influenza, tuberculosis, and diarrhea/enteritis. We adapted our environment to address these illnesses, proving that we have intuition and knowledge to address the causes of premature death. When it comes to lifestyle diseases we can start by looking at the actions that cause illness to exist in the body. Our bodies can deal with a lot. One unhealthy meal won't cause harm, however the impact of eating unhealthy meals repeatedly over the course of years will. To reverse the damage we must focus on diet and lifestyle. By identifying the patterns that lead to disease we can also look into the patterns that promote health and vitality in our bodies.

We are currently at a major crossroads: the direction of abundance & convenience and the direction of access & willingness. We live in a world where we desire can be delivered to our doorstep in less than a day, and whatever we want to eat can be ordered, purchased, and consumed without much thought. This world of convenience allows us to focus on other things in life, and gives us the freedom to partake in more leisurely activities.

We also live in a world of access and willingness. Where if we want to, we can purchase organic food, buy holistic remedies, and partake in wellness practices. However we must be willing, and even if it is inconvenient we do it because we know the value and we can obtain it.

I do not believe that people would choose to live an unhealthy life, and if you choose that path, this book isn't for you. It is my view that most people simply don't know where to begin when it comes to proper self-care. My goal with this book is to give you a place to start. This book should not be the only resource you use, but one of many you discover along your health journey.

WHO AM I WRITING THIS BOOK FOR?

This book was written for two people. First, the everyday person. We all have an innate desire to be healthy. We wish to be strong in a healthy body free of disease, pain, and aliments. We crave the energy level to live our lives to the fullest. Without the proper fuel and habits we will not be able to achieve these goals.

This book is meant to offer you 101 healthy habits that will start you on the path to live a healthier lifestyle today. Some habits are easier than others, so even the most reluctant person can start from the easiest place. For the health conscious person you can learn or relearn a new habit or improve upon one you already follow.

The goal is to establish a new habit and make it part of your lifestyle. Once one habit is achieved, you will take on another. These habits are meant to help aid your body in healing, detoxification, and nourishment. I hope you enjoy discovering a habit you currently engage in to validate that practice, and then discover a new habit that you can implement to continue down the journey of health and healing.

Second is for my fellow wellness providers. This book is for your clients. As a wellness provider I understand the struggle of client compliance. We offer our clients the best solutions to help them with their health concerns - we write it out, spell it out in detailed steps, and follow-up with sessions. When we learn that the client hasn't taken any of the recommended actions we often blame ourselves, and think poorly of our clients. Being frustrated we continually look for methods, tricks, and new agreements for them to take on the actions we prescribe. What we learn is that in order for someone to change, the level of desperation must be high enough for new behaviors to emerge. Sadly, it can take a health crisis to finally move the client into the appropriate actions and habits they need to implement to save their life.

This book is for you to offer them new ideas on where they can start. The best place to start is where they are in life. Have them find a habit they are already implementing, and help them validate why that habit is a positive step forward. Then work with them to start to implement more habits they can work on.

It's going to be up to all of us to help heal our fellow human. We become healers because we see what's possible for those around us and we found a way to help our fellow man. And woman. The hardest part is convincing people we have a way that can help. My hope is that this book will be one of the ways you can help your community.

HOW TO USE THIS BOOK:

Step 1: Identify a health habit you are currently doing.
Step 2: Congratulate yourself that you are doing something positive towards your health.
Step 3: Learn if there are adjustments / improvements you can make to your current health habit.
Step 4: Identify a new health habit you want to take on.
Step 5: Practice implementing that habit.
Step 6: Once you've mastered that habit see Step 2.

How this book is written:

This book is categorized into three parts: Lifestyle | Nutrition | Fitness. These health habits were inspired by three forms of sciences; Chinese, Ayverada, and Modern.

I divide each habit into three sections:

1 – Why it's important
2 – The science behind it
3 – How to do it

This book is designed to be a resource and reference guide for your health journey. You are encouraged to skip around and identify a health habit that is important to you and start there. Be inspired with the implementation of that new habit.

Remember some habits are not daily habits, but the things you do instead of another behavior. For instance, you might find the use of ghee inspiring and beneficial, but you won't necessarily replace all other kinds of fats with ghee, but simply add ghee to the rotation of foods in your diet.

How Habits Form:

According to the Webster's dictionary a habit is a "behavior pattern acquired by frequent repetition or physiologic exposure that shows itself in regularity or increased facility of performance."

In his book, *The Power of Habit*, Charles Duhigg, explores the science behind habit creation and reformation.

The main concepts Duhigg develops in his book are the habit loop, the golden rule habit, and the keystone habit.

The Habit loop: This is a neurological pattern that governs any habit. It consists of three elements: a cue, a routine, and a reward. Understanding these components can help in understanding how to change bad habits or form good ones. The habit loop always starts with a cue, a trigger that transfers your brain into a mode that automatically determines which habit to use. The heart of the habit is a mental, emotional, or physical routine. Finally there is a reward, which helps your brain determine if this particular loop is worth remembering for the future.

The Golden rule of habit is a rule to follow that will help you stop your addictive habits and replace them with new ones. It states that if you keep the initial cue, replace the routine, and keep the reward, change will eventually occur, although individuals who do not believe in what they are doing will likely fall short of the expectations and give up. Belief is a critical element of such a change, though it can be structured in a number of ways including group settings. Often people who join groups like accountability groups are better off than those who act alone. A keystone habit is an individual pattern that is unintentionally capable of triggering other habits in the lives of people. If you start with a small habit it will eventually lead to other habit changes in the future.

Habits form both consciously and unconsciously and can be learned and unlearned.

When we look at someone's success we can learn about their achievement through the habits they have taken to get there. In the context of health we can glean from habits of healthy, productive, energized people and breakdown their daily and weekly habits so we can achieve a similar result.

The challenge here is that most people will compare the results of years of accumulation with a certain habit to the results of a new habit in the making. When a similar result isn't accomplished it can be quickly abandoned because it didn't work, we didn't see the results quickly enough, and we allow frustration to overwhelm us. When we feel frustrated, we are in the presence of uncomfortable emotions. Who wants to be surrounded by their uncomfortable emotions? The person that wants results. We've all heard the saying, life begins outside our comfort zone. Being outside our comfort zone results in feeling discomfort, frustration, boredom, and confusion. We can spend our entire lives avoiding these emotions and never learn how to deal with the growth that comes from this uncomfortable place.

If adults got their secondary set of teeth at age 20 we would be a toothless society because we would not want to deal with the pain that goes with it. However, because of education and other people surviving the pain, we teach our children that going through pain is normal, natural, and part of the process. Once it grows out it no longer hurts.

The same goes for any habit you want to learn and adopt. Ask someone who has adapted that habit into their life and you will hear, it was painful, uncomfortable, and sometimes it hurt, but eventually I learned and it no longer hurt. In fact it got easier and more fun.

There are three things to know about why habits form whether you like it or not.

1. Signal speed. 2. Willpower muscle. 3. Autopilot.

The average brain is made up of 40% gray matter and 60% white matter.

White matter lays under the gray matter and is composed of long nerve fibers insulated by myelin sheets. Myelin is the fatty tissue that makes white matter white. It is one of the reasons that people are good at things. As you repeat an action the neurons associated with that action wrap that action in myelin. Every time you put in an hour of practice you earn yourself another wrap in myelin around the neuron associated with that activity. More myelin means the nerve impulse can travel more quickly and efficiently across the axons. This means the action can be done more easily and skillfully, and will require less concentration. A bare unmyelined neuron will have a speed of 2mph, while the signal speed of a fully developed myelin neuron is about 200mph. Practice makes perfect because practice makes myelin, myelin makes perfect. This is the major principle in the Talent Code.

Author Daniel Coyle explains that athletes, singers, and performers that we would describe as talented are actually incredibly diligent individuals. They have put in hours and hour of practice, until their brains are packed with myelin associated with their craft. Regardless of whether you have developed an unconscious bad habit (bite finger nails) or a good habit (drink enough water throughout the day) our brains are doing the same thing to make that action easier. Athletes put so much concentration into perfecting their sports it becomes an automatic habit.

The second thing to know about habit formation is willpower. By the 1980s the theory that willpower is a learnable skill had been widely accepted. It was thought that willpower can be taught the same way we teach children how to do math and say thank you.

In *The Power of Habits*, Duhigg talks about how a group of Ph.D students totally changed our existing view on willpower. If willpower is a learnable skill how can we be diligent on one day and binge watch a TV show on others? That would be like forgetting to ride a bike every other day.

The amount of willpower we have is finite and, like a muscle, you can tire it out if you work it too hard. When we resist the cookie we have less fuel in our willpower tank, leading us to give in when faced with another choice, and feel frustrated more easily.

Another experiment was conducted where participants needed to conduct a four month money management system. This required them to keep detailed logs, and avoid going to the movies or eating out. What they found was that, people's finances improved as they progressed through the program. As people strengthened their willpower muscles in one part of their lives, they also smoked fewer cigarettes, drank less alcohol and caffeine, ate less junk food and were more productive at work and school. Once willpower became stronger, it touched every area of their lives.

The third thing to know about habits is to build your autopilot. In the 1990s neurologists figured out a way to get sensors into rats' brains. This study showed that after doing the same task over and over again the brain that was once heightened will fall asleep doing the task.

A task-bracket or 'chunking' pattern of neuronal activity emerges when a habit is formed, wherein neurons activate when a habitual task is initiated, show little activity during the task, and reactive when the task is completed.

Your brain is taking a series of actions and grouping them into a single task, making the process require less conscious effort. The part of the brain responsible for this is the bal ganglia. When we try to start walking, we bring our arms up, slowly lift our foot up, shift our weight, and repeat with the other leg. We don't think of these as separate behaviors now, but when we learn something new, we practice those behaviors and then chunk them together.

Habits need a cue in order for it kick-in in and autopilot the task. For example it's the morning alarm that triggers the morning jog. When we are focusing on a new task, we unconsciously do habits we don't know we are doing. For example, when I get bored I find myself checking Facebook. It happens so fast before I realize it, and think – hey this isn't what I wanted to do. To identify your cue is figuring out what your cue is, i.e. thinking of a certain phase for a sentence. Habit phases can be anything from feeling bored or frustrated to the clock striking 3:00 p.m.

How do you build a habit?

We have all heard the saying that it takes 21 days to incorporate a new habit in your life.

In doing research for this book I learned that the 21 day habit number came from a plastic surgeon back in the 1950s named Maxwell Maltz.

When Dr. Maltz would perform an operation — like a nose job, for example — he found that it would take the patient about 21 days to get used to seeing their new face. Similarly, when a patient had an arm or a leg amputated, Maltz noticed that the patient would sense a phantom limb for about 21 days before adjusting to the new situation.

These experiences prompted Maltz to think about his own adjustment period to changes and new behaviors, and he noticed that it also took him about 21 days to form a new habit. Maltz wrote about these experiences and said, "These, and many other commonly observed phenomena tend to show that it requires a minimum of about 21 days for an old mental image to dissolve and a new one to jell."

In 1960, Maltz published that quote and his other thoughts on behavior change in a book called Psycho-Cybernetics. The book went on to become a blockbuster hit, selling more than 30 million copies.

It makes sense why the "21 Days" myth would spread. It's easy to understand. The time frame is short enough to be inspiring, but long enough to be believable. And who doesn't like the idea of changing your life in just three weeks?

But the problem is that Maltz was simply observing what was going on around him and wasn't making a statement of fact. Furthermore, he made sure to say that this was the minimum amount of time needed to adapt to a new change.

On average, it takes more than two months before a new behavior becomes automatic, 66 days to be exact. How long it takes a new habit to form varies widely depending on the behavior, the person, and the circumstances.

Phillippa Lally is a health psychology researcher at University College London. In a study published in the European Journal of Social Psychology, Lally and her research team decided to figure out just how long it actually takes to form a habit.

The study examined the habits of 96 people over a 12-week period. Each person chose one new habit for the 12 weeks and reported each day on whether or not they did the behavior and how automatic the behavior felt.

Some people chose simple habits like "drinking a bottle of water with lunch." Others chose more difficult tasks like "running for 15 minutes before dinner." At the end of the 12 weeks, the researchers analyzed the data to determine how long it took each person to go from starting a new behavior to automatically doing it.

In Lally's study, it took anywhere from 18 days to 254 days for people to form a new habit. In other words, if you want to set your expectations appropriately, the truth is that it will probably take you anywhere from two months to eight months to build a new behavior into your life, not 21 days.

Interestingly, the researchers also found that "missing one opportunity to perform the behavior did not materially affect the habit formation process." In other words, it doesn't matter if you mess up every now and then. Building better habits is not an all-or-nothing process.

Embracing the longer timeline can help us realize that habits are a process and not an event. Believing that it only takes 21 days can set you up for failure, thinking that once you get to the 21st day you no longer need to work on the habit. Habits never work that way and you have to embrace the process and commit to the system.

Understanding this from the beginning makes it easier to manage your expectations and commit to making small, incremental improvements

— rather than pressuring yourself into thinking that you have to do it all at once.

To start there are habit tracking apps but they can get cumbersome because you have to develop the habit of tracking the new habit on an app. That's two new habits you'll need to develop.

To simplify, utilize already existing cues to develop a new habit. You can use new cues to create new habits, or use old cues to replace bad habits with good ones.

For example, new habit, meditate for 20 minutes. Cue, after I brush my teeth I go into meditation. Existing habit of buying a cookie after lunch, replaced with a new habit of buying a cup of tea after lunch. New habit, studying every night, cue finish dinner or shower, then study. Being consistent with your cue is particularly important.

All you need is the right cue and the right mindset when building the habit. A growth mindset teaches us that new connections are growing in our brain and things will get easier if you persist.

Whatever habit you choose to start with, start with one. When you feel like you've mastered it i.e you are doing it without thinking about it, and it becomes part of your day, you are ready for a new habit.

101 Health Habits to choose from:

- Lifestyle
- Nutrition
- Fitness

Lifestyle:

1. Acupuncture
2. Breathing Before Eating: parasympathetic (relaxed) state

3. Breathe Outdoors
4. Buy Fresh, Buy Local
5. Buying Organic
6. Chiropractor
7. Cry
8. Dry Brush Massage
9. Earthing
10. Energy Healing
11. Fast
12. Go To The Beach
13. Give Gratitude
14. Cultivate Healthy Relationships
15. Make Your Own Beauty Products
16. Homemade Cleaning Supplies
17. House Plants
18. Hug
19. Journal
20. Laugh
21. Learn
22. Get A Massage
23. Meditate
24. Be in Nature
25. Oil Pulling
26. Create Positive Affirmations
27. Make Quality Friendships
28. Reduce Your Food Waste
29. Rest and Relax
30. Rotate Your Diet
31. Sleep
32. Smile More
33. Take a Bath
34. Tongue Scraping
35. Warm Your Food on the Stove

Nutrition:

1. Almonds
2. Apple Cider Vinegar
3. Asparagus
4. Avocados
5. Basil
6. Beets
7. Bone Broth
8. Brussel Sprouts
9. Carrots
10. Cauliflower
11. Celery
12. Coconut flour
13. Coconut Oil
14. Cod Liver Oil
15. Dark Chocolate
16. Eggs
17. Garlic
18. Ghee
19. Ginger
20. Go Booze Free
21. Goji Berries
22. Grass-fed Butter
23. Grass-fed Calves Liver
24. Grass-fed Cheese
25. Green Tea
26. Honey
27. Kefir
28. Kimchi
29. Kombucha
30. Leafy Greens
31. Lemons

32. Mushrooms
33. Nutritional Yeast
34. Olive Oil
35. Onions
36. Free-Range Chicken
37. Oysters
38. Pink Himalayan Salt
39. Pumpkins
40. Pumpkin Seeds
41. Raw Milk
42. Rosemary
43. Sage
44. Make Your Own Salad Dressing
45. Sardines
46. Sauerkraut
47. Sea Vegetables
48. Soaked Nuts
49. Sprouts
50. Squash
51. Tomatoes
52. Turmeric
53. Water
54. Wild Caught Salmon

Exercise:

1. Bike
2. Grow a Garden
3. High Intensity Training
4. Go on a Hike
5. Martial Arts
6. Olympic Lifting
7. Qigong
8. Squatting
9. Go For a Walk
10. Resistance Training
11. Yoga

1. ACUPUNCTURE

The Why:

Acupuncture is based upon the Eastern philosophy of chi (also spelled qi), which is the Chinese term for the life force or vital energy that animates all living things. In traditional Chinese medicine chi flows through pathways in the body known as meridians. Illness results from the flow of chi through the meridians being blocked, or when the two types of chi (yin and yang) are out of balance. Acupuncture is the practice of placing thin needles at acupuncture points, which are said to coincide with points at which meridians cross, to improve the flow and restore the balance of chi.

The Science:

Results from a number of studies[1] suggest that acupuncture may help ease types of pain that are often chronic such as low back pain, neck pain, and osteoarthritis/knee pain. It also may help reduce the frequency of tension headaches and prevent migraine headaches. Therefore, acupuncture appears to be a reasonable option for people with chronic pain to consider.

The effects of acupuncture on the brain and body and how best to measure them are only beginning to be understood. Current evidence suggests that many factors—like expectation and belief—that are unrelated to acupuncture needling may play important roles in the beneficial effects of acupuncture on pain.

[1] "Acupuncture: In Depth," National Center for Complementary and Integrative Health (U.S. Department of

Health and Human Services, February 21, 2017), https://nccih.nih.gov/health/acupuncture/introduction#hed3.

The How:

If you decide to visit an acupuncturist, check his or her credentials. Most states require a license, certification, or registration to practice acupuncture; however, education and training standards and requirements for obtaining these vary from state to state. Although a license does not ensure quality of care, it does indicate that the practitioner meets certain standards regarding the knowledge and use of acupuncture. Most states require a diploma from the National Certification Commission for Acupuncture and Oriental Medicine for licensing. Ask the practitioner about the estimated number of treatments needed and how much each treatment will cost. Some insurance companies may cover the costs of acupuncture, while others may not.

2. BREATHE BEFORE EATING: BEING IN A PARASYMPATHETIC (RELAXED) STATE

The Why:

Imagine if you could actually control your body's ability to digest, metabolize and assimilate food. Well you can, it's called getting yourself into a parasympathetic (relaxed) state before enjoying your delicious meal. This breaks down the nutrients in our food so we can absorb them and receive their full health benefits.

The Science:

The parasympathetic system conserves energy while it slows the heart rate down, increases intestinal activity, opens the blood vessels and allows us to take those deep, calming breaths. When it comes to improving our digestive wellness, the parasympathetic nervous system is where it begins.[2]

The How:

Bring yourself to your body, sitting there at the table. Be committed to being fully present. Begin breathing with the intention of relaxing and achieving the goal of being nowhere else. This is the fastest way to shift our bodies into a more relaxed state.

Step 1: Take five deep breaths.
Step 2: Smell your food.
Step 3: chew slowly.
Step 4: Count to 30 while chewing.
Step 5. Swallow.

[2] "Psychology of Eating," Psychology of Eating, accessed September 26, 2019, http://psychologyofeating.com/secret-digestive-wellness/.

Life happens so fast. It deserves our full attention and eating deserves it's full due. Relax. Enjoy the process. There's no good reason to move so fast that we can't metabolize our meal. Health is not about speed, it's all about slow.

3. BREATHE OUTDOORS

The Why:

Get out and breathe some fresh air. The amount of serotonin in your body is greatly affected by the amount of oxygen you inhale. Serotonin can significantly lighten your mood and promote a sense of happiness and well-being. Fresh air will leave you feeling more refreshed and relaxed.

The Science:

Research shows that spending time in fresh air, surrounded by nature, increases energy in 90% of people. "Nature is fuel for the soul", according to Richard Ryan, researcher and professor of psychology at the University of Rochester. "Often when we feel depleted we reach for a cup of coffee, but research suggests a better way to get energized is to connect with nature."

The How:

1. Go outside.
2. Lie on the ground or sit with your back straight.
3. Inhale deeply, pulling in as much air as you can using your diaphragm.
4. Exhale fully but not forcefully; simply let the breath go.
5. Repeat inhales and exhales for 30 to 40 rounds with your own rhythm.
6. On the last round, exhale and then hold your breath until your body feels the need to breathe.
7. Inhale deeply, then hold your breath for 10 seconds.
8. Repeat steps 3–6 for three or four rounds.[3,4]

[3] Shelby Stanger, "Change Your Breath, Change Your Life," Outside Online, August 13, 2019,

https://www.outsideonline.com/2086911/iceman-cometh.

[4] Richard M. Ryan et al., "Vitalizing Effects of Being Outdoors and in Nature," Journal of Environmental

4. BUY FRESH, BUY LOCAL

The Why:

Local food is known for its freshness. The produce is harvested when ripe and thus fresher and more flavorful than food that comes from further away. When making your food choices, whether it be at a restaurant or grocery store, buy fresh & buy local. Your money stays within the community and the local farmers get more financial support when their customers buy directly from them.

The Science:

When you buy local food you reduce your carbon footprint by contributing less to pollution from transportation. A study from the National Resources Defense Council (NRDC) has the proven numbers showing that non-local food, especially imported food, makes up a larger and larger percentage of Americans' diets, and has a much higher emissions impact than locally produced food.

Approximately 950 cases of asthma, 16,870 missed schools days, 43 hospital admissions, and 37 premature deaths could be attributed to the worsened air quality from food imports.

The How:

The key to eating locally is knowing what's in season. Research guides to learn the natural flow of fruits and vegetables throughout the year. Cooking seasonally can be a big adjustment at first, but the deprivation of certain fruits and vegetables for months at a time only makes them taste better when you finally have them, fresh and full of in-season flavor.

Psychology 30, no. 2 (2010): pp. 159-168,
https://doi.org/10.1016/j.jenvp.2009.10.009.

Small local farmers often use organic methods but sometimes cannot afford to become certified organic. Visit a farmer's market and speak with the farmers to find out what methods they use.[5]

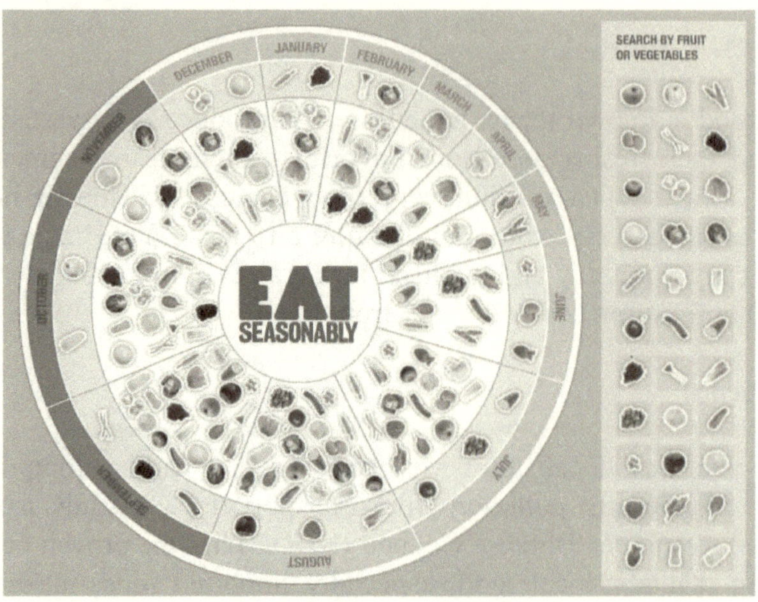

[5] California Air Resources Board, "Sustainable Freight Transport," California Air Resources Board, accessed October 2, 2019, https://ww3.arb.ca.gov/gmp/sfti/sfti.htm.

5. BUYING ORGANIC

The Why:

How your food is grown or raised can have a major impact on your mental and emotional health as well as the environment. Organic foods often have more beneficial nutrients, such as antioxidants, than their conventionally-grown counterparts. People with allergies to foods, chemicals, or preservatives often find their symptoms lessen or go away when they eat only organic foods.

One of the big benefits of eating organic is you lessen your exposure to pesticides. Chemicals such as fungicides, herbicides, and insecticides are widely used in conventional agriculture and residues remain on (and in) the food we eat.

The Science:

A number of studies have been completed regarding the effects of antioxidants from organic foods on overall health, and the predominant results have shown that antioxidants tend to have more of an impact when they come from organic foods. This may be due to the fact that foreign chemicals are not negatively interacting with the different vitamins, minerals, and organic compounds that are so essential for the positive impact of fruits and vegetables in the prevention of cancer, heart diseases, premature aging, vision problems, and cognitive malfunction. Recent research suggests that choosing organic food can lead to increased intake of nutritionally desirable antioxidants and reduced exposure to toxic heavy metals.
The How:

Buy in season – Fruits and vegetables are cheapest and freshest when they are in season. Find out when produce is delivered to your market so you're buying the freshest food possible.

Shop around – Compare the price of organic items at the grocery store, the farmers' market and other venues (even the freezer aisle).

Remember that organic doesn't always equal healthy. Making junk food sound healthy is a common marketing ploy in the food industry but organic baked goods, desserts, and snacks are usually still very high in sugar, salt, fat, or calories. It pays to read food labels carefully.

6. CHIROPRACTOR

The Why:

Chiropractic is based on the notion that the relationship between the body's structure (primarily that of the spine) and its function (as coordinated by the nervous system) affects health. Essentially, the basic principle upon which the entire profession is built is that the body has the amazing, innate ability to heal itself (under the right conditions), and it is the chiropractor's job to help create an environment to facilitate this. Because the nervous system controls every cell and organ in your body, chiropractors focus their attention on the health of your spine being properly aligned and, if there are shifts, helping the spine come back into alignment.

The Science:

Researchers have studied spinal manipulation for a number of conditions ranging from back, neck, and shoulder pain to asthma, carpal tunnel syndrome, fibromyalgia, and headaches. Much of the research has focused on low back pain, and has shown that spinal manipulation appears to benefit some people with this condition.

A 2010 review of scientific evidence on manual therapies for a range of conditions concluded that spinal manipulation/mobilization may be helpful for several conditions in addition to back pain, including migraine and cervicogenic (neck-related) headaches, neck pain, upper- and lower-extremity joint conditions, and whiplash-associated disorders. The review also identified a number of conditions for which spinal manipulation/mobilization appears not to be helpful (including asthma, hypertension, and menstrual pain) or the evidence is inconclusive (e.g., fibromyalgia, mid back pain, premenstrual syndrome, sciatica, and temporomandibular joint disorders).

The How:

- Ask about the chiropractor's education and licensure.
- Mention any medical conditions you have, and ask whether the chiropractor has specialized training or experience in the condition for which you are seeking care.
- Ask about typical out-of-pocket costs and insurance coverage. (Chiropractic is covered by many health maintenance organizations and private health plans, Medicare, and state workers' compensation systems.)
- Tell the chiropractor about any medications (prescription or over-the-counter) and dietary supplements you take. If the chiropractor suggests a dietary supplement, ask about potential interactions with your medications or other supplements.
- Tell all of your health care providers about any complementary health approaches you use. Give them a full picture of what you do to manage your health. This will help ensure coordinated and safe care.

7. CRY

The Why:

Tears actually help relieve stress. This is because emotional tears are responsible for the release of the stress hormone cortisol produced in the body. A good cry has been known to help people feel better even when the problems persist and the reasons for crying are still relevant.

The Science:

Allow yourself to have a good cry. A study performed by Dr. William H. Frey II at the St Paul-Ramsey Medical Centre found that stress-related tears and tears caused by physical irritants (think chopping an onion) are not one and the same. Tears that are provoked by stress help your body rid itself of nasty chemicals that raise cortisol (the stress hormone). In other words: you'll feel a whole lot better after the emotional downpour passes.

Crying does not only cleanse us mentally, it can cleanse our body too. Tears that are produced by stress help the body get rid of chemicals that raise cortisol, the stress hormone. A study conducted by Dr. William H. Frey II, a biochemist and director of the Psychiatry Research Laboratories at St. Paul-Ramsey Medical Centre, found like other exocrine processes, including exhaling, urinating, and sweating, toxic substances are released from the body when we cry. Several of the chemicals present in emotional crying are the protein prolactin, adrenocorticotropic hormones, and the endorphin leucine-enkephalin, which reduces pain.

The How:

Letting the Tears Flow

- Find a good place to cry. Most people who have trouble letting themselves cry prefer to experience their emotions alone.
- Clear your head of distractions
- Think deeply about what's making you sad
- Let your emotions swell until you cry[6],
- Feel better

[6] Paul Chernyak and Lpc, "How to Cry and Let It All Out," wikiHow (wikiHow, May 18, 2019), http://www.wikihow.com/Cry-and-Let-It-All-Out.

8. DRY BRUSH MASSAGE

The Why:

The skin is the largest elimination organ. One-third of impurities in the body are excreted through the skin. Dry brushing removes dead layers of skin and opens pores. It also stimulates hormones, circulation, and oil producing glands.

Proponents of the technique claim dry brushing stimulates the lymphatic system, unclogs pores, exfoliates dead skin cells, reduces cellulite, and basically gives you the skin of your dreams.

The Science:

The lymphatic system is a major part of the body's immune system. It is made up of organs and lymph nodes, ducts and vessels that transport lymph throughout the body. Many of these lymph vessels run just below the skin and proponents of dry brushing claim that brushing the skin regularly helps stimulate the normal lymph flow and the body to detoxify itself naturally.

The How:

First you'll need a high-quality dry brush. Look for one with bristles made from natural materials. They should feel stiff but not overly so. Ideally, choose a brush with a long handle so you can reach your entire back and other hard-to-reach spots.

Dry skin brushing should be done daily for best results, or even twice a day if you like. Try incorporating it into your normal daily routine, such as doing your brushing before your morning shower and then again after work (avoid doing it too close to bedtime, as it may leave you feeling energized).

When brushing, always brush toward your heart, which is best for circulation and your lymphatic system. You can brush your entire body (including the soles of your feet). Start at your feet and work your way up your legs to your arms, chest, back, and stomach. Avoid brushing your face (unless you have a special brush designed for this delicate skin), your genitals, or any areas with irritations or abrasions (including varicose veins).

The pressure you apply while brushing your skin should be firm but not painful (avoid "scrubbing"). Your skin should be pink after a session (not red or irritated) and you can brush for as long (or as little) as you would like. An average dry brushing session may last between two and 20 minutes.[7]

[7] Katie Wells et al., "Dry Brushing for Skin: Benefits & How to Do It the Right Way," Wellness Mama®,

July 30, 2019, https://wellnessmama.com/26717/dry-brushing-skin/.

9. EARTHING

The Why:

Healing with Earthing aka grounding. When we go barefoot we come in contact with the free electrons from the Earth's surface. Studies have proven that this practice improves blood pressure, reduces cortisol, and improves sleep.

The Science:

There have been some studies associating earthing during sleep with health benefits – in general, leading to reduced levels of pain and lower levels of the stress hormone cortisol.

Grounding can have a positive effect on mood.

Subjective reports that walking barefoot on the earth enhances health and provides feelings of well-being can be found in the literature and practices of diverse cultures from around the world.
One study reports that free or mobile electrons from the earth can resolve chronic inflammation by serving as natural antioxidants.

Another study found that test subjects reported improved sleep, reduced stress and decreased pain. It was reported that grounding the human body during sleep reduced night-time levels of cortisol and enhanced the circadian rhythm.[8]

[8] Gaétan Chevalier et al., "Earthing: Health Implications of Reconnecting the Human Body to the Earth's

Surface Electrons," Journal of environmental and public health (Hindawi Publishing Corporation, 2012), https://www.ncbi.nlm.nih.gov/pmc/articles/PMC3265077/#B13.

The How:

Earthing can be done in two ways:

1. Direct physical contact with the earth. For example, walking barefoot on grass or swimming in the ocean.
2. Using Earthing mats. These can be used under your arms or feet while on a computer to reduce the amount of EMFs you are exposed to.

Experts tend to encourage the use of earthing mats over spending time outside, claiming that it's impossible to spend enough time in connection with nature while still leading a modern lifestyle.[9]

[9] Ashingu et al., "Health Benefits Of Earthing Grounded In Science?," Critical Cactus, August 13, 2015,

http://www.criticalcactus.com/health-benefits-of-earthing-grounded-in-science/.

10. ENERGY HEALING

The Why:

Energy healing is a holistic practice that activates the body's subtle energy systems to remove blocks. By breaking through these energetic blocks, the body's inherent ability to heal itself is stimulated.

Various ancient cultures used different modalities to stimulate the body's natural ability to heal, seeing internal energy as a powerful force of good. Reiki is the Japanese tradition of energy healing, and it dates back to the early 20th century. Chakras, the seven energy transmission centers of the body, are described in ancient Hindu texts.

The Science:

New York Presbyterian Hospital/Columbia University Campus conducted one of the first studies ever performed to determine the effectiveness of Reiki treatments on the autonomic nervous system. This blind, random study included a Reiki treatment group, a "sham" treatment group and a "control" group. The testing began with all participants at "baseline" autonomic nervous systems levels. The results within the Reiki treatment group showed a lowering of these levels including heart rate, respiration and blood pressure. These positive results led the team to recommend further, larger studies to look at the biological effects of Reiki treatment.

The How:

Your left hand is the hand used for receiving energies. You output energies through the right hand if you wish to transfer energies to another person.

1.   Raise your left hand palm upward.

2. Visualize white healing energy flowing into your palm and along your arm.

3. Visualize further, the white light traveling first down to your feet and spiraling upward through your main energy centers red through violet.

4. Visualize the energy then traveling throughout your body and cleansing every part of you.

5. Send any collection of negative energies that you intuitively perceive to be present, back out into the universe, exiting through the blue energy center at the throat.

6. Feel yourself revitalized by further intake of love/light intelligent energy through the left palm.

7. Intuitively know when you have received sufficient healing energy and stop the process.[10]

[10] Green Lotus, "Reiki Really Works: A Groundbreaking Scientific Study," GreenLotus, 2011, https://www.uclahealth.org/rehab/workfiles/Urban Zen/Research Articles/Reiki_Really_Works-A_Groundbreaking_Scientific_Study.pdf.

11. FAST

The Why:

Give your digestion system a break and build ketones in your body, which is our fat burning mode. Fasting has been shown to improve eating patterns, hunger signals, and brain function.

The Science:

Intermittent fasting changes the function of cells, genes and hormones. When you don't eat for sustained periods of time, several things happen in your body. Your body initiates important cellular repair processes that change hormone levels to make stored body fat more accessible.

Here are some of the changes that occur in your body during fasting:

Insulin levels: Blood levels of insulin drop significantly, which facilitates fat burning.

Human growth hormone: The blood levels of growth hormone may increase as much as five-fold. Higher levels of this hormone facilitate fat burning and muscle gain.

Cellular repair: The body induces important cellular repair processes, such as removing waste material from cells.

Gene expression: There are beneficial changes in several genes and molecules related to longevity and protection against disease.

The How:

Here are three ways to practice" intermittent fasting:

1. Fast and feast regularly: Fast for a certain number of hours, then consume all calories within a certain number of hours. Practice this two to three times x per week.
2. Eat normally, then fast one to two times per week: Consume your normal meals every day, then pick one or two days a week where you fast for 24 hours. For example, eat your last meal Sunday night, and then don't eat again until dinner the following day.
3. Fast occasionally: probably the easiest method for the person who wants to do the least amount of work. Simply skip a meal whenever it's convenient. On the road? Skip breakfast. Busy day at work? Skip lunch. Eat poorly all day Saturday? Make your first meal of the day dinner on Sunday.[11,12]

[11] Steve Kamb, "Intermittent Fasting For Beginners: Should You Skip Breakfast?," Nerd Fitness, July 31,

2019, https://www.nerdfitness.com/blog/a-beginners-guide-to-intermittent-fasting/.

[12] Leonie K Heilbronn et al., "Alternate-Day Fasting in Nonobese Subjects: Effects on Body Weight, Body

Composition, and Energy Metabolism," The American journal of clinical nutrition (U.S. National Library of Medicine, January 2005), https://www.ncbi.nlm.nih.gov/pubmed/15640462.

12. GO TO THE BEACH

The Why:

Our feet have more sweat glands & nerve endings per centimeter than any other part of the body. When we go to the beach and put our feet in the sand and ocean we absorb some much needed nutrients. Sea water contains high level of the minerals our bodies need for healing and detoxifying like magnesium, potassium and iodine.

The Science:

Minerals already dissolved in water are more bioavailable than solid forms, although many factors affect absorption within the small intestine, such as pH levels, health of the mucosal lining and the presence of other nutrients, as noted in the text, "Advanced Nutrition and Human Metabolism." A French study published in a 2002 edition of the "European Journal of Clinical Nutrition" found that the absorption and bioavailability of magnesium in magnesium-rich mineral water was almost 60% in healthy male volunteers.

The How:

How to enjoy alone time on the beach:

Stay hydrated.
Protect your skin from overexposure.
Pack an umbrella.
Read a book.
Make a beach playlist.
Put your feet in the sand and water.
Go on a walk.
Enjoy the water.[13]

13 wikiHow, "How to Have Fun at the Beach," wikiHow (wikiHow, March 29, 2019),

13. GIVE GRATITUDE

The Why:

Gratitude increases mental strength. We all have the ability and opportunity to cultivate gratitude. Rather than complain about the things you think you deserve, take a few moments to focus on all that you have. Developing an "attitude of gratitude" is one of the simplest ways to improve your satisfaction with life. Recognizing all that you have to be thankful for even during the worst times fosters resilience.

The Science:

Research has shown gratitude not only reduces stress, but it may also plays a major role in overcoming trauma. A 2006 study published in Behavior Research and Therapy found that Vietnam War veterans with higher levels of gratitude experienced lower rates of post-traumatic stress disorder. A 2003 study published in the Journal of Personality and Social Psychology found that gratitude was a major contributor to resilience following the terrorist attacks on September 11.

http://www.wikihow.com/Have-Fun-at-the-Beach.

The How:

Keep a gratitude journal. Establish a daily practice in which you remind yourself of the gifts, grace, benefits, and good things you enjoy. Setting aside time on a daily basis to recall moments of gratitude associated with ordinary events, your personal attributes, or valued people in your life gives you the potential to interweave a sustainable life theme of gratefulness.[14,15]

[14] Amy Morin, "7 Scientifically Proven Benefits of Gratitude," Psychology Today (Sussex Publishers),

accessed September 27, 2019, https://www.psychologytoday.com/blog/what-mentally-strong-people-dont-do/201504/7-scientifically-proven-benefits-gratitude.

[15] Robert Emmons, University of California, and University of California, "10 Ways to Become More

Grateful," Greater Good, accessed September 27, 2019, http://greatergood.berkeley.edu/article/item/ten_ways_to_become_more_grateful1/.

14. CULTIVATE HEALTHY RELATIONSHIPS

The Why:

Being in a healthy relationship makes you healthier. When you witness the interaction of loving couples holding hands you experience the love they have for one another. Holding hands is a merging of the yin & yang energy and part of healing. Being in love has been proven to boost our immune system.

The Science:

A happy marriage may also speed the rate that wounds heal, according to a 2005 study at Ohio State University. It found that a married couple's 30-minute positive, supportive discussion sped up their bodies' ability to recover from an injury by at least one day. [16,17]

The How:

Keep an open line of honest communication.
Be faithful.
Be supportive.
Put the couple first.
Brag on each other
Have fun together.
Don't forget you are your own person.

[16] "Healthy Relationships," Loveisrespect.org, accessed September 27, 2019,

http://www.loveisrespect.org/healthy-relationships/.

[17] "Eight Simple Rules For A Happy Marriage," Pure Romance | Inspire, July 2, 2019,

https://www.pureromance.com/inspire/buzzworthy/eight-simple-rules-for-a-happy-marriage.

15. MAKE YOUR OWN BEAUTY PRODUCTS

The Why:

Exposing our bodies to synthetic chemicals has similar negative effects as those we experience when we eat non-organic foods. They are poisons that cause our immune systems to become damaged and inflamed. This inflammation response creates free radicals called oxidants which destroy cells. The more cells you lose the more your skin shrinks and folds, causing wrinkles.

Homemade beauty products contain extracts of different ingredients such plants, oils and fruits. These ingredients soothe, tone, moisturize and heal your skin and hair. This practice means you know exactly what you are putting into your body and can control what your skin absorbs.

The Science:

Your skin is your largest organ, absorbing up to 60% of what you put on it. Yet 80%of the ingredients that are used in daily personal care products have never been tested for safety. The laws governing the cosmetics industry date back to 1938 and haven't shifted since. The average American woman puts between 12 and 20 chemicals on their skin 365 days a year through shampoo, soap, lotion, cosmetics, etc.

The European Union has banned 1,300 chemicals that are used as ingredients in beauty products. The US has only banned 11.

The How:

There are 7 basic ingredients in making your own homemade beauty products:

1. Coconut Oil
2. Shea Butter
3. Cocoa Butter
4. Beeswax
5. Liquid Carrier Oil
6. Arrowroot Powder
7. Essential Oils

Homemade Lotion Recipe:

INGREDIENTS
1/2 cup almond oil or jojoba oil (or any other liquid oil)1/4 cup coconut oil
1/4 cup beeswax
1 tsp vitamin E oil (optional)
2 TBSP shea butter or cocoa butter (optional) essential oils, vanilla extract, or other natural extracts to suit your preference (optional)

Combine almond oil (or any other liquid oil), coconut oil, and beeswax in a double boiler or a glass bowl on top of a pot of boiling water. If using shea or cocoa butter, add it here.
As the water heats, the ingredients will start to melt. Stir occasionally to incorporate.
When all ingredients are completely melted, add vitamin E oil (if using) and any essential oils or scents like vanilla.
Pour into whatever jar or tin you will use for storage. Small mason jars work perfectly for this. (I like to use 8 ounce jars like these.)

Note: This will not pump well in a lotion pump!

Use as you would regular lotion. This lotion is ultra-moisturizing and more oily than water-based lotions so you won't need to use as much. It also has a longer shelf life than some homemade lotion recipes since all ingredients are already shelf stable and no water is added. Use within 6 months for best moisturizing benefits.[18]

Note: This will not pump well in a lotion pump!

18 Katie Wells, "Homemade Lotion Recipe," WellnessMama, September 5, 2018, https://wellnessmama.com/3765/homemade-lotion-recipe/.

16. HOMEMADE CLEANING SUPPLIES

The Why:

Synthetic household products contain harmful chemicals that react with the ozone from the air, creating toxins like formaldehyde. The inside of your home contains approximately two to five times as many common chemical pollutants as areas outside of homes, according to the Environmental Protection Agency.

Indoor pollutants can cause headaches, flu-like symptoms, neurological issues and possibly increase the risk of respiratory disease.

Natural cleaning products are therefore better for both your health and the environment. Buying natural cleaning products helps to support green companies, but if cost is an issue people can still participate in eco-friendly cleaning practices by making homemade cleaners.

The Science:

Studies have shown that using a household cleaning spray, even as little as once a week, raises the risk of developing asthma.

Currently, government regulations don't require ingredients to be listed on any cleaning products.

The How:

Use natural products for cleaning and disinfecting. Make homemade cleaners with simple ingredients such as vinegar, club soda and baking soda.
To make an all-purpose cleaner, fill spray bottles with:
- 1/4 cup baking soda
- 1/2 cup vinegar
- 1/2 gallon water

17. HOUSE PLANTS

The Why:

Get yourself a few house plants and you will have a direct source of the oxygen we need to breath. According to a study out of Texas A&M (*year)* Plants are also linked to productivity,and having plants at home and at work increases memory retention and concentration.

The Science:

In the great outdoors, plant roots tap the groundwater table for water which then evaporates through its leaves in a process known as transpiration. Studies show that this accounts for about 10% of the moisture in the atmosphere. The same thing happens at home (minus the groundwater table part), which increases the humidity indoors. While this may sound unappealing during hot moist months, it's a gift during drier months or if you live in an arid climate. According to Bayer Advanced, studies at the Agricultural University of Norway document that using plants in interior spaces decreases the incidence of dry skin, colds, sore throats and dry coughs. And other research reveals that higher absolute humidity is conducive for decreased survival and transmission of the flu virus.[19]

[19] "5 Benefits of Houseplants," Bioadvanced, accessed September 27, 2019, https://www.bayeradvanced.com/articles/5-benefits-of-houseplants.

The How:

Pick plants that suit your tastes and willingness to work. Pay attention to how much light is necessary for the plants you pick so you can make sure to have a suitable place in your apartment or home for them.

If you travel a lot choose easy care plants, i.e. those that do not require a lot of care and watering. This way you can go away without worrying or having to hire a house sitter.

A lot of houseplants can leave their indoor safety in the summer for the porch in the front yard, but make sure it's summer before you put them outside. Before you bring them back indoors in the fall, be sure to check for any pests hitching a ride under the leaves, on the stems or on the soil surface. [20,21]

[20] Melissa Breyer, "5 Health Benefits of Houseplants," TreeHugger (Treehugger, August 29, 2019),

http://www.treehugger.com/health/5-health-benefits-houseplants.html.

[21] "Choosing The Best Plants For Your Indoor Containers," Gardening Know How, April 5, 2018,

https://www.gardeningknowhow.com/houseplants/hpgen/determining-the-best-plants-for-your-indoor-containers.htm.

18. HUG

The Why:

There is a saying by Virginia Satir, a respected family therapist, "We need four hugs a day for survival. We need eight hugs a day for maintenance. We need twelve hugs a day for growth."
Hugging is an organic way of interacting with one another. We all have felt the deep the need for a big hug.

The Science:

Research shows that hugging and laughter is extremely effective at healing sickness, disease, loneliness, depression, anxiety and stress.

A proper deep hug, where the hearts are pressing together, can benefit you in these ways:

1. The nurturing touch of a hug builds trust and a sense of safety. This helps with open and honest communication.
2. Hugs can instantly boost oxytocin levels, which heal feelings of loneliness, isolation, and anger.
3. Holding a hug for an extended time lifts one's serotonin levels, elevating mood and creating happiness.
4. Hugs strengthen the immune system. The gentle pressure on the sternum and the emotional charge this creates activates the Solar Plexus Chakra. This stimulates the thymus gland, which regulates and balances the body's production of white blood cells, which keep you healthy and disease free.

The How:

1. Hug like you mean it. Hugging some people is like embracing a telephone pole.
2. Be willing to be vulnerable. Open your arms.
3. Close your eyes.
4. Breathe into the embrace.
5. Lean into the embrace.
6. Squeeze, but don't suffocate.
7. Just BE with the person you're embracing.
8. Let go.

19. JOURNAL

The Why:

This is a mental exercise that helps you get out of your head, process your thoughts, record a history of your mental state, and boosts your memory & comprehension. It's a great practice to write down what you think about to give your thoughts a place to go.

The Science:

A report by the University of Victoria noted that "Writing as part of language learning has a positive correlation with intelligence."

Journaling is an exploration of language, you'll have the natural urge to search for new words and increase your vocabulary. The report goes on to say, "One of the best single measures of overall intelligence as measured by intelligence tests is vocabulary."[22]

The How:

Reflect on how you are currently feeling and how you want to feel.
Take a moment to go within and listen to how you're feeling. Put this on paper. Do you feel tired? Do you feel stressed? Do you feel happy? Are you excited?

Now write down how you want to feel today. Do you want to feel liberated? Connected? Energetic? Patient?
Reflect on what you can do to help you feel the way you want to feel today.[23]

[22] Reza Falahati, "The Relationship Between Students' IQ and Their Ability to Use Transitional Words and Expressions in Writing," accessed October 2, 2019, http://journals.uvic.ca/index.php/WPLC/article/viewFile/5160/2132.

[23] Naomi Arnold, "7 Journal Writing Prompts for Beginners," The Huffington Post (TheHuffingtonPost.com,

20. LAUGH

The Why:

Laughter is the best medicine. Find people that make you laugh and spend time with them. For me those people are my family and close friends. There is strong evidence that laughter can actually improve health and help fight disease.

The Science:

Laughter, along with an active sense of humor, may help protect you against a heart attack, according to a recent study by cardiologists at the University of Maryland Medical Center in Baltimore. The study, which is the first to indicate that laughter may help prevent heart disease, found that people with heart disease were 40% less likely to laugh in a variety of situations compared to people of the same age without heart disease.

The How:

Laugh Deeply

When you laugh, put your hand on your diaphragm and feel it. When you practice laughter in the future, make sure you can feel it deep in your body. Treating laughter as an exercise will keep your funny muscles strong. Practice laughing with a wide grin and a deep belly chuckle.[24,]

December 7, 2017), http://www.huffingtonpost.com/naomi-arnold/7-journal-writing-prompts_b_5934252.html.

[24] Klare Heston, "How to Laugh," wikiHow (wikiHow, June 6, 2019), http://www.wikihow.com/Laugh.

21. LEARN

The Why:

Never stop learning. Educating yourself on how to be, and stay, healthy is an ongoing process. Learning can come from books, podcasts, seminars, experts, self-experimentation etc. It's important in a healthy lifestyle to continually grow and expand your knowledge.

The Science:

Brains operate on the "use it or lose it" principle. There's a reason that you forget how to speak a language or work out a trigonometry problem. This is due to the weakening of neural pathways over time, causing you to lose information in the brain that isn't used regularly.

Research has found that the brain generates more cells than it needs, with those that receive chemical and electrical stimuli surviving and the rest dying off. The brain has to receive regular stimulation to a given pathway in the brain to sustain those cells, which is why lifelong learning is so important to brain health.

The How:

Studies have shown that for a student to learn and retain information like historical events, vocabulary words, or science definitions, it's best to review the information one to two days after first studying it. One theory is that the brain actually pays less attention during shorter learning intervals. So repeating the information over a longer interval, say a few days or a week later rather than in rapid succession, sends a stronger signal to the brain that it needs to retain the information.

One way to signal to the brain that information is important is to talk about it. Teaching someone else what you just learned helps you reinforce what you are learning. Other techniques that solidify learning are self-testing and writing down information on flashcards.[25,26]

[25] "The 10 Biggest Breakthroughs in the Science of Learning," Brainscape Blog, May 26, 2017,

https://www.brainscape.com/blog/2012/10/breakthroughs-science-of-learning-2/.

[26] Tara Parker-Pope, "Better Ways to Learn," The New York Times (The New York Times, October 6,

2014), https://well.blogs.nytimes.com/2014/10/06/better-ways-to-learn/?_r=0.

22. GET A MASSAGE

The Why:

Self-love and massage go hand in hand. Pun intended. Getting a massage has been shown to lower anxiety, improve digestion, and result in a better night's sleep.

The Science:

The massage research study has shown on a cellular level that massage therapy helps the body heal. Even after one session, the body starts to respond to massage therapy. Researchers did blood and muscle tests on individuals before and after a vigorous workout; one group received massage therapy after exercise and the other group did not. The 'after massage' results surprised researchers. The post-massage blood and muscle tissue showed an increase in a gene responsible for mitochondria development. The mitochondria are known for cell growth and energy production. The lifting and kneading of muscle tissue common in the Swedish and deep tissue techniques were shown to 'turn off' genes associated with inflammation.

The How:

Give a Better Partner Massage

Use your body weight so you don't get tired. Good massage is less about your grip and more about your stance and the use of gravity.

Have your partner sit on the floor on a pillow while you sit on the couch or in a chair while you stand behind her. They can also lie on the floor on some blankets or a mat, but sitting allows for extra stretching by leaning forward as you massage their back.

Don't forget the oil. To prevent uncomfortable friction and help your hands glide easily, use some lotion or a little bit of olive oil when massaging. Don't just pour it on their back, use the oil on your own hands and warm them up.

Do no harm. Avoid pinching or grabbing muscles. You can prevent this by keeping your fingers together and using your whole hand in the massage. With a massage, use soft strokes to warm up the muscles before you try to knead them.

At the start, ask if the pressure is enough. They should feel pressure, but not pain. Adjust as needed: If they want a deeper massage, lean in further, using your body weight. You can also use your knuckles to target really stiff muscles.[27,28,29,30]

27 Admin, "The Science behind Massage: Why Does It Work?," Athletico, May 23, 2019,

http://www.athletico.com/2013/01/09/the-science-behind-why-massage-works/.

28 Gisela Telis, "Massage Mystery Mechanism," Sciencemag.org, February 2012, sciencemag.org.

29 Roni Rabin, "Regimens: Massage Benefits Are More Than Skin Deep," New York Times, September 2010.

30 "How Do I Give Better Massages?," Lifehacker, accessed September 27, 2019,

http://lifehacker.com/5871832/how-do-i-give-better-massages.

23. MEDITATE

The Why:

Meditation is the heartbeat of a nourishing & healthy lifestyle. It calms you down, relaxes your body, sharpens your thinking and has other fantastic health benefits. Find your practice: guided, breathing cycles, one word focus, letting go of thoughts, etc. Like working out does for your body, meditation serves to strengthen the mind.
The Science:

A study conducted in 1984 found that those who meditate regularly are more perceptive than those who do not. In short, the researchers found that meditation practitioners needed a shorter period of time to register and recognize stimuli than their non-meditating counterparts.

Another study found that meditation helps to increase your creativity. Researchers at Leiden University in The Netherlands found that certain forms of meditation open up your mind to new ideas. This isn't in the abstract. What it means is that your internal censor is less active after certain forms of meditation, allowing you to fully realize ideas that you might otherwise shut down before they fully blossom.

The How:

Simple meditation for beginners:

- Sit or lie comfortably. You may even want to invest in a meditation chair.
- Close your eyes.
- Make no effort to control the breath; simply breathe naturally.
- Focus your attention on the breath and on how the body moves with each inhalation and exhalation. Notice the movement of your body as you breathe. Observe your chest, shoulders, rib cage, and belly. Simply focus your attention on your breath without controlling its pace or intensity. If your mind wanders, return your focus back to your breath.
- Maintain this meditation practice for two to three minutes to start, and then try it for longer periods.[31,32]

[31] Gaiam, "Meditation 101: Techniques, Benefits, and a Beginner's How-To," Gaiam, accessed

September 27, 2019, http://www.gaiam.com/discover/158/article/meditation-101-techniques-benefits-and-a-beginners-how-to.

[32] Jared R Lindahl et al., "A Phenomenology of Meditation-Induced Light Experiences: Traditional

Buddhist and Neurobiological Perspectives," Frontiers in psychology (Frontiers Media S.A., January 3, 2014), https://www.ncbi.nlm.nih.gov/pmc/articles/PMC3879457/.

24. BE IN NATURE

The Why:

Shake off the city and get yourself into nature. Being in nature automatically instills a sense of calm, helps put things into perspective, and heightens our senses. You can always find a peaceful spot to think, contemplate, and relax.

The Science:

Getting outside can improve your eye health. Really this should count for a big reason:

Preventing Computer Vision Syndrome (CVS), the term used to describe eye problems caused by staring at a screen close to your face for prolonged periods. If you work on a computer for a living and watch TV when you're not working, this puts you at risk of developing the symptoms associated with CVS: blurred vision, double vision, dry/red eyes, eye irritation, headaches, and neck or back pain.

Getting outside and focusing on objects more than two feet from your face can help to prevent and even reverse these symptoms.

The How:

Being in nature requires the simple choice of going outside, finding some green space, and enjoying the outdoor environment. It can be as simple as finding a city park, or as complex (and exciting) as planning your vacation to a national park. The point is to make it into a daily habit in your lifestyle.[33]

[33] "Find a Park (U.S. National Park Service)," National Parks Service (U.S. Department of the Interior),

accessed September 27, 2019, https://www.nps.gov/findapark/index.htm.

25. OIL PULLING

The Why:

Oil pulling is a powerful detoxifying Ayurvedic technique that has recently become a very popular remedy for many different health ailments. It is an oral detox that helps cure tooth decay, boost the immune system, and whiten teeth.

The Science:

The increasing interest surrounding oil pulling in the general public has correspondingly increased scientific interest in the practice. One study showed that oil pulling with sesame oil can boost overall oral health by significantly reducing Streptococcus mutans, a microbe that contributes to tooth decay. Some scientists believe the lipids in the oil reduce the adhesion of bacteria to the teeth and gums, possibly explaining its bacteria-diminishing effects.

The Journal of Ayurveda and Integrative Medicine, for example, recently highlighted a study that reviewed holistic approaches to oral health and discovered that oil pulling is one of the most effective natural health solutions known to scientists that prevent tooth decay and loss. Praised for curing more than 30 systemic diseases, the authors of this study have some profound things to say about this ancient natural healing practice.

The How:

1. Make sure to oil pull first thing in the morning right after you get out of bed, before you brush your teeth or drink anything.
2. Gently swish 1 – 2 tablespoons of coconut oil in your mouth and between your teeth for 10-20 minutes making sure that you don't swallow any of the oil. (Do this gently so you don't wear out your jaw and cheeks!)
3. Spit out the oil in the trash and immediately rinse your mouth out with warm water (use salt water for added antimicrobial properties).
4. Finally, brush your teeth as normal.[34]

[34] Josh Axe, "Coconut Oil Pulling Is the New Flossing (It Stops Tooth Decay, Prevents Cavities, Kills Bad Breath & More!)," Dr. Axe, June 2, 2018, https://draxe.com/oil-pulling-coconut-oil/.

26. CREATE POSITIVE AFFIRMATIONS

The Why:

We choose our beliefs so we might as well choose ones that create a beautiful life. You are grounded by what you believe. Believe that you are amazing, incredible, and loved. Because you are.

The Science:

Research from Carnegie Mellon University provides the first evidence that self-affirmation can protect against the damaging effects of stress on problem-solving performance.

"An emerging set of published studies suggest that a brief self-affirmation activity at the beginning of a school term can boost academic grade-point averages in underperforming kids at the end of the semester. This new work suggests a mechanism for these studies, showing self-affirmation effects on actual problem-solving performance under pressure," said J. David Creswell, assistant professor of psychology in CMU's Dietrich College of Humanities and Social Sciences.

The How:

Choose one negative thought you have about yourself and write down the positive opposite that counteracts that belief.

Example:
Negative Thought: "They'll never like me."
Underneath it is I am not confident enough to approach an attractive person at a bar.

Positive Thought: "They'll love me!"
Underneath that thought is, I have some intelligent things to share, I wonder if that attractive person would like to have a conversation? Let's find out.

Make your affirmations short so they're easier for you to remember.

Start your affirmations with "I" or "My." ...
Write your affirmations in the present tense.[35]

[35] S. Renee Smith, "How to Write Your Own Affirmations," dummies, accessed September 27, 2019,

http://www.dummies.com/health/mental-health/self-esteem/how-to-write-your-own-affirmations/.

27. MAKE QUALITY FRIENDSHIPS

The Why:

Having a solid group of friends actually increases your pain tolerance. It all has to do with endorphins. Endorphins are our body's natural painkillers. They're a part of the brain's pleasure and pain circuits, and they promote bonding. It is theorized that social interactions trigger endorphin release in the brain, lending to the "feel-good" positive emotions and happiness when we see our friends. We link this strong, feel-good effect with the fact that endorphins are powerful painkillers to believe that having close friendships may actually prove to be more effective than morphine when in pain.

The Science:

Researchers took a look at social lives of the elderly and noticed a very important finding. Changes in their social lives, such as smaller and interconnected social networks, less social support and dwindling community event attendance were classified as evidence for cognitive decline. As cognition becomes more impaired, people can't keep up with their usual circle of friends anymore and instead receive social support from family members or just withdraw from their community.

A positive find in this study was that men who were classified with mild cognitive impairment or dementia reported that with their diagnoses, they felt even more encouragement and support from their spouses. Additionally, men started to socialize 15% more than before.

That being said, maintaining friend groups keeps your mind young and fresh, and their support can actually benefit you more if you start on a mental decline as you age.

The How:

One of the easiest ways to make new friends is compatibility. Find people interested in some of the same things you are. When talking to new people mention music you enjoy, ask about how they spend their time, bring up a new sport / class / book you have been wanting to dive into and see what they say.

Besides being a companion for activities, the best of friends also need to provide emotional support. This is often where friends and best friends divide. As you get to know someone, you want to know if they have the same values as you. Remember it's always best to listen five times more than you speak when providing emotional support.[36,37]

36 "Learn How to Make Friends As An Adult Using These 5 Steps," Science of People, January 30, 2019,

http://www.scienceofpeople.com/2016/07/the-science-of-friendship/.

37 "Learn How to Make Friends As An Adult Using These 5 Steps," Science of People, January 30, 2019,

http://www.scienceofpeople.com/2016/03/how-to-make-friends/.

28. REDUCE YOUR FOOD WASTE

The Why:

Food waste is a worldwide epidemic, and it's well past time the average person started fighting back. More than one-third of all food produced globally is wasted or spoiled. Americans throw away up to 40% of the food they buy, and organic matter in landfills provides 20% of all methane emissions, a potent greenhouse gas that contributes considerably to climate change.

The Science:

The environmental impact of food waste is growing. About 70% of our water and 50% of our land is devoted to agriculture. So when we do not eat that food, it's a huge unnecessary use of resources. About 33 million cars' worth of greenhouse gases are produced to grow food that never gets eaten.

The How:

Shop smart and realistically.
When cooking, don't overprepare food.
Save – and actually eat – leftovers.
Store food in the right places.
Avoid clutter in your fridge, pantry and freezer.
Treat expiration and sell-by dates as guidelines.

29. REST AND RELAX

The Why:

Taking time in the day to relax gives your body the time to recover andrest, and in turn lowers your cortisol levels. However, there is a difference between relaxation and laziness. Relaxation is the intentional practice to allow your body to recover. Laziness is the purposeful act of avoiding work.

The Science:

When faced with numerous responsibilities and tasks, or the demands of an illness, relaxation techniques may take a back seat in your life. But that means you might miss out on the many health benefits of relaxation.

Practicing relaxation techniques can reduce stress symptoms by:

- Slowing your heart rate.
- Lowering blood pressure.
- Slowing your breathing rate.
- Reducing activity of stress hormones.
- Increasing blood flow to major muscles.
- Reducing muscle tension and chronic pain.
- Improving concentration and mood.
- Lowering fatigue.
- Reducing anger and frustration.
- Boosting confidence to handle problems.

The How:

There are several main types of relaxation techniques, including:

1. *Autogenic relaxation.* Autogenic means something that comes from within you. In this relaxation technique, you use both visual imagery and body awareness to reduce stress. You repeat words or suggestions in your mind to relax and reduce muscle tension. For example, you may imagine a peaceful setting and then focus on controlled, relaxing breathing, slowing your heart rate, or feeling different physical sensations, such as relaxing each arm or leg one by one.

2. *Progressive muscle relaxation.* In this relaxation technique, you focus on slowly tensing and then relaxing each muscle group. This helps you focus on the difference between muscle tension and relaxation, and become more aware of physical sensations. One method of progressive muscle relaxation is to start by tensing and relaxing the muscles in your toes and progressively work your way up to your neck and head. You can also start with your head and neck and work down to your toes. Tense your muscles for at least five seconds and then relax for 30 seconds, and repeat.

3. *Visualization.* In this relaxation technique, you form mental images to take a visual journey to a peaceful, calming place or situation. During visualization, try to use as many senses as you can, including smell, sight, sound and touch. For instance, If you imagine relaxing at the ocean, think about the smell of salt water, the sound of crashing waves and the warmth of the sun

on your body. You may want to close your eyes, sit in a quiet spot and loosen any tight clothing.[38]

38 "Relaxation Techniques: Try These Steps to Reduce Stress," Mayo Clinic (Mayo Foundation for

Medical Education and Research, April 19, 2017), http://www.mayoclinic.org/healthy-lifestyle/stress-management/in-depth/relaxation-technique/art-20045368?pg=1.

30. ROTATE YOUR DIET

The Why:

This practice helps you get all the nutrients you need from food. We are designed to eat a variety of different plants and proteins to give us the 100+ vitamins & minerals our body needs.

In addition, the rotation diet is a helpful tool in identifying sensitivities, and may help prevent new food allergies from developing.

The Science:

Rotation dieting to reduces the stress-load of food exposure called nomenclature. There are so many foods that are closely related - broccoli, cabbage, canola, asparagus all belong to the same family-we can easily become overexposed to the same proteins. When we begin to understand and classify food groups, we can better incorporate more variety into our diets and minimize consistent exposure to the same food.

The How:

Meal planning is essential because it helps you keep track of what you're eating from day to day.

Here are three ways of thinking about rotating your diet.

1. Think about the foods you typically eat every day. On your meal plan, put those foods on the first, fourth, and seventh day of the week. Then fill in other things for the remaining days.
2. Think of colors. Take pictures of your plate and count how many colors you have eaten throughout the week.
3. Name as many vegetables as you can. Write them down. Make a game of preparing a vegetable using two different recipes for each. Go through your entire list and score yourself with how many you eat each month.[39]

39 Barbara Faison et al., "Benefits of a Rotation Diet," Real Food Real Deals, May 17, 2019,

http://realfoodrealdeals.com/benefits-rotation-diet/.

31. SLEEP

The Why:

The quality of sleep we get is reflective of the quality of our lifestyle. When we get good, deep and consistent quality sleep this reflects back into our waking life a healthier lifestyle. i.e. quality nutrition, proper stress management, ability to do physical exercise, etc.

Embrace your need for sleep! Lack of sleep can lead to weight gain, chronic fatigue, and loss of productivity.

The gold standard in sleep is when we can answer yes to the following questions:

- Ability to go to lay in bed without looking at a screen.
- Ability to fall asleep quickly.
- Ability stay asleep (except if you wake up to pee).
- Ability to wake up refreshed without an alarm.
- Ability to remember your dreams.
- Ability to remember if your dreams are pleasant.

The Science:

Sleep experts know that the mental clarity lost because of a few sleepless nights can often be restored with just one good night's rest. Now, UT Southwestern Medical Center researchers have identified a key molecular mechanism that regulates the brain's ability to mentally compensate for sleep deprivation.

The relationship of circadian rhythms to sleep is relatively well understood. Continuing studies in genetics and molecular biology promise further advances in our knowledge of how the circadian clock works and how a succession of behavioral states adapt to changes in light/dark cycles. In addition to the circadian component, there is a fundamental regulatory process involved in programming sleep. Consider that the longer an individual remains awake, the stronger the desire and need to sleep becomes. This pressure to sleep defines the homeostatic component of sleep. The precise mechanism underlying the pressure that causes us to feel a need to sleep remains a mystery. What science does know is that the action of nerve-signaling molecules (neurotransmitters) and of nerve cells (neurons) located in the brainstem and at the base of the brain determines whether we are asleep or awake. Additionally, there is recent evidence that the molecule adenosine (composed of the base adenine linked to the five-carbon sugar ribose) is an important sleepiness factor: it appears to "keep track" of lost sleep and may induce sleep. Interestingly, caffeine binds to and blocks the same cell receptors that recognize adenosine. This suggests that caffeine disrupts sleep by binding to adenosine receptors and preventing it from delivering its fatigue signal. The homeostatic regulation of sleep helps reinforce the circadian cycle. We usually sleep once daily because the homeostatic pressure to sleep is hard to resist after about 16 hours, and then while we sleep, our closed eyes block the light signals to the biological clock.

The How:

Develop a "sleep hygiene" ritual before bed.

- Stick to a regular schedule. The body loves ritual.
- Go to bed and wake up around the same time each day.
- 15 to30 min before bedtime do one of the following:

- *Meditate* (Use a guided meditation if you are unfamiliar how to meditate). This will help you rest your adrenal glands, aka stress organ, so you can better manage stress during the day.
- *Gratitude Journal* (Write down 5 things you were grateful that happen that day). This will give you added perspective and focus on attracting more of those grateful moments.
- *Take a cold shower.* Start with warm water and then let your body be drenched in cold water for 30 seconds at the end. This will naturally stimulate your immune system.

- Create a relaxing bedroom environment conducive to consistent quality sleep.
-

- Set temperature to 68 degrees.
- Have a heavy blanket that has a little weight on top of your body.
- Block out any natural light coming in from the window. The darker the better.[40,41]

[40] "Molecule Helps Sleep-Deprived Rebound Mentally," ScienceDaily (ScienceDaily, February 25, 2009),

https://www.sciencedaily.com/releases/2009/02/090224132908.htm.

[41] James Clear, "Get Better Sleep: How to Fall Asleep Fast and Beat Sleep Deprivation," James Clear,

October 24, 2018, http://jamesclear.com/better-sleep.

32. SMILE MORE

The Why:

Studies suggest that smiling, forced or not, can have a positive effect on your mood and make you better looking.

Smiles are pretty darn attractive for more reasons than one. A smile suggests that you are personable, easygoing, and empathetic. In fact, a study in the European Journal of Social Psychology found that smiling actually makes you more attractive to those you smile at.

The Science:

Smiling can help you manage stress and anxiety by releasing endorphins, chemicals that make you happier. Endorphins are the same chemicals you get from working out or running, resulting in what is known as a runner's high. Smiling even makes your immune system stronger by making your body produce white blood cells to help fight illnesses. One study found that hospitalized children who were visited by story-tellers and puppeteers who made them smile and laugh had higher white blood cell counts than those children who did not receive visits.

The How:
- Spend time with friends and family who are most likely to cheer you up.
- Take time out and watch a film or a TV show you find funny.
- Even when you don't feel like it, try and force yourself to smile – you may find that a forced smile becomes genuine.
- Reflect on happy memories by looking through photographs.[42]

42 András Béres et al., "'Does Happiness Help Healing?" Immune Response of Hospitalized Children May

33. TAKE A BATH

The Why:

Sometimes our bodies need for rest & self-love is greater than making sure you don't miss a workout. Taking a bath lets your adrenals rest so your cortisol (stress hormone) doesn't need to fire. Too much cortisol in the body can hinder weight loss efforts.

The Science:

In 2002 a University of Wolverhampton study found that a daily bath, usually at the end of the day, significantly improved the mood and optimism of the participants. These results were attributed to a combination of bodily comfort, warmth, isolation, and body positioning.

It turns out that our bodies associate horizontal conditions with relaxation and vulnerability, particularly in the bath, which possibly mimics the warm, liquid conditions of the womb. Some scholars think that this particular positioning gives us a sensation of security.[43]

Change during Visits of the Smiling Hospital Foundation's Artists," Orvosi hetilap (U.S. National Library of Medicine, October 23, 2011), https://www.ncbi.nlm.nih.gov/pubmed/21983400.

[43] Bryony Gordon, "In Hot Water? Have a Bath and Relax," The Telegraph (Telegraph Media Group, .

October 14, 2002), http://www.telegraph.co.uk/news/health/alternative-medicine/4711987/In-hot-water-Have-a-bath-and-relax.html.

The How:

1. If you'd prefer, take a quick shower beforehand to cleanse your skin and wash your hair so that you don't feel like you're bathing in dirt. Then, step out and start prepping!

2. Give your tub a scrub and rinse away any residue left over from shampoo, body wash and even stray strands of hair! Begin filling your tub with lukewarm to hot water, but be sure the temperature isn't scalding. Not only is this bad for your skin, but it can make you feel dizzy while laying in the bath. Test the water with your elbow before getting in.

3. As the water is running, add in 10 to15 drops of your favorite essential oils for a soothing scent that will put your body and mind at ease.

4. Just before stepping in, set the atmosphere by lighting some of your favorite candles, playing some soothing tunes and grabbing a book or magazine. As tempting as it may be to have your phone nearby, don't. Let yourself unplug for a while.

5. As the water starts to cool down, turn the faucet and let some hot water run to reheat the tub. Hot baths are known to reduce cramps, headaches and even help with the sniffles.

6. Once you're ready to lather up, use your favorite body wash to keep skin clean and moisturized. Then let the water drain and give yourself a quick rinse in the shower to wash away any remaining soap. Once finished, carefully step out onto the floor mat and pat your body dry. Then apply a full body moisturizer to keep your skin hydrated and you're good to go![44]

[44] Diana Crisan, "How To Take A Bath," Makeup.com (Makeup.com, March 5, 2019),

https://www.makeup.com/how-to-take-a-bath.

34. TONGUE SCRAPING

Tongue Scraping is an Ayurvedic self-care ritual for oral hygiene that removes bacteria, food debris, fungi, toxins, and dead cells from the surface of the tongue. When we sleep, our digestive system remains awake, removing toxins from our body by depositing them onto the surface of our tongue. If we don't scrape away these toxins, they are reabsorbed by the body and can lead to respiratory difficulties, digestive problems, and a compromised immune system.

The Science:

Dental research has concluded that a tongue scraper is more effective at removing toxins and bacteria from the tongue than a toothbrush. Although brushing and flossing will loosen and move debris around, they do not actually remove the bacteria. Almost half of our oral bacteria live on and in the deep crevices of our tongue; the scraping action of a tongue scraper collects these toxic tongue coatings, which can range in color from clear, white, yellow, or green, and removes them from the body.

The How:

This Ayurvedic daily routine for maintaining oral health should be done on a regular basis, in the morning upon rising, and on an empty stomach. A tongue scraper is a long, thin, flat piece of metal that is bent in a "U" shape.

Standing in front of a mirror, you scrape your tongue by simply holding the two ends of the scraper in both hands, sticking out your tongue, and placing the scraper as far back on your tongue as possible. With firm but gentle pressure, scrape the surface of your tongue in one long stroke. Rinse the scraper and repeat (usually 5 to 10 times) until your tongue feels clean and is free of coating.[45]

[45] Vinícius Pedrazzi et al., "Tongue-Cleaning Methods: a Comparative Clinical Trial Employing a

Toothbrush and a Tongue Scraper," Journal of periodontology (U.S. National Library of Medicine, July 2004), https://www.ncbi.nlm.nih.gov/pubmed/15341360.

35. WARM YOUR FOOD ON THE STOVE AKA DITCH THE MICROWAVE

The Why:

Microwaving cooks food at very high temperatures in a very short amount of time. This results in a great deal of nutrient loss for most foods, especially vegetables.

The Science:

One study by Dr. Hans Hertel explored how microwaves change the molecular structure of food and the effects of that food on the human body. In his study, he found that individuals who consumed the microwaved foods experienced a decrease in HDL cholesterol, and a reduced red and white blood cell count.

The How:

Prepare your meals in advance so that you always have a good meal available on those days when you're too busy or too tired to cook.

For example, take your dinner out of the freezer the morning or the night before you plan to eat it so you don't end up scrambling to defrost a five-pound chunk of beef two hours before dinnertime. Make soups and stews in bulk, and then freeze them in gallon-sized freezer bags or other containers. An hour before meal time, just take one out and defrost it in a sink of water until it's thawed enough to slip into a pot, then reheat it on the stove.

A toaster oven makes a GREAT faux-microwave for heating up leftovers! Keep it at a low temperature — around 200 to 250 degrees F — and gently warm a plate of food over the course of 20 to 30 minutes.

36. ALMONDS

The Why:

Almonds are among the world's best sources of vitamin E, with just one ounce providing 37% of the recommended daily intake. Getting plenty of vitamin E from foods is linked to numerous health benefits.

The Science:

Vitamin E is the name for a group of fat soluble antioxidants. These antioxidants tend to build up in cell membranes in the body, protecting the cells from oxidative damage.

Several studies have linked higher vitamin E intake with lower rates of heart disease, cancer and Alzheimer's disease

The How:

 Look for raw organic almonds. Eating them raw is good, however eating them soaked is best because it provides more their e nutrients.[46]

[46] Donielle, "How to Soak Almonds," Natural Fertility and Wellness, February 26, 2019,

http://www.naturalfertilityandwellness.com/how-to-soak-almonds/.

37. APPLE CIDER VINEGAR

The Why:

Having a bottle of Apple Cider Vinegar is a staple in any health nut's home. Apple cider vinegar increases stomach acid which improves digestion and nutrient assimilation by increasing HCl production.

The Science:

Apple Cider Vinegar in its raw form is an excellent digestive tonic. It's so rich in living enzymes that it helps to break food down to its bare components, making it far easier to assimilate. The acetic acid present in Apple Cider Vinegar has also been shown to help with mineral absorption, enabling us to get the most out of the foods we eat.[47,48]

The How:

Drinking a glass of water mixed with a 1 to3 teaspoons of apple cider vinegar15 to20 minutes before a meal can improve digestion and nutrient assimilation by increasing HCl production. Start with 1 teaspoon to see how you fare, and go from there.
Swish about 4 more ounces of water and swallow it to prevent the acid from affecting tooth enamel and irritating the esophagus.

Be sure to use raw, unpasteurized apple cider vinegar with the mother.

[47] J Kashimura, M Kimura, and Y Itokawa, "The Effects of Isomaltulose, Isomalt, and Isomaltulose-Based

Oligomers on Mineral Absorption and Retention," Biological trace element research (U.S. National Library of Medicine, September 1996), https://www.ncbi.nlm.nih.gov/pubmed/8909697.

[48] Tomoo Kondo et al., "Vinegar Intake Reduces Body Weight, Body Fat Mass, and Serum Triglyceride

Levels in Obese Japanese Subjects," Bioscience, biotechnology, and biochemistry (U.S. National Library of Medicine, August 2009), https://www.ncbi.nlm.nih.gov/pubmed/19661687.

38. ASPARAGUS

The Why:

Asparagus contains a unique array of phytonutrients. Like chicory root and Jerusalem artichoke, it is an important source of the digestive support nutrient, inulin. Asparagus is an excellent source of vitamin K, folate, copper, selenium, vitamin B1, vitamin B2, vitamin C, and vitamin E. It is a very good source of dietary fiber, manganese, phosphorus, vitamin B3, potassium, choline, vitamin A, zinc, iron, protein, vitamin B6, and pantothenic acid. Additionally, it is a good source of magnesium and calcium.

Science:

Recent research has underscored the value of careful storage of fresh asparagus. The key scientific finding here involves respiration rate. Like all vegetables, asparagus doesn't instantly "die" when it is picked, but instead, continues to engage in metabolic activity. This metabolic activity includes intake of oxygen, the breaking down of starches and sugars, and the releasing of carbon dioxide. The speed at which these processes occur is typically referred to as "respiration rate." Compared to most other vegetables, asparagus has a very high respiration rate. At 105 milligrams of carbon dioxide released per six minutes per 100 grams of food (at a refrigerator temperature of 41°F/5°C), this rate is about five times greater than those of onions and potatoes (stored at a room temperature of 68°F/20°C), and about three times greater than those of leaf lettuce and ripe avocado (stored at a refrigerator temperature of 41°F/5°C) . Asparagus' very high respiration rate makes it more perishable than its fellow vegetables, and also much more likely to lose water, wrinkle, and harden.

The How:

Buy fresh, organic asparagus, and look for bright green or violet-tinged spears. Spears should be straight, firm, and uniformly-sized, with closed (not flowering) tips. Ideally, buy fresh asparagus on the day that you plan to use it. Asparagus is one of the first green vegetables to come into season at the end of winter. Fresh, American-grown asparagus often appears in stores in late February, but the vegetable is at its best – and is usually cheapest – in April and May.

Store asparagus in a refrigerator or on ice. Use asparagus within two or three days of purchase, and preferably sooner. If you do need to keep it for a day or two, the best way to preserve the spears is to place them upright in a bowl (or even a small vase) of cold water. You can wrap the ends of the spears in a damp paper towel and refrigerate them in a plastic bag for up to three days.

39. AVOCADO

The Why:

Avocados are nature's miracle fruit. They contain more potassium than bananas, are loaded with essential fatty acids and beyond delicious.

The Science:

Recent studies analyzed the overall impact of avocado on the average U.S. diet, with some fascinating results. In one broad-based, national study, participants who reported eating any amount of avocado over a 24 hour period were compared to participants who reported eating no avocado during that same time period. The avocado-eating U.S. adults were found to have greater fiber intake (over 6 grams more for the day); greater potassium intake (439 milligrams more); greater vitamin K intake (57 micrograms more); and greater vitamin E intake (2.2 milligrams more) than U.S. adults who ate no avocado. It is worth adding that U.S. adults consuming avocado also averaged 43 milligrams more magnesium, 5.6 grams more monounsaturated fat, and 3.2 grams more polyunsaturated fat. The study authors also noted that avocado eating was associated with better overall diet quality, as well as better intake of vegetables and fruits as a whole.

The How:

Easy guacamole recipe

INGREDIENTS
3 medium avocados or 4 small ones;
1 firm tomato, finely diced;
1/2 white onion;
1/2 cup chopped cilantro;
2 tbsp fresh lemon or lime juice;
Optional salt and pepper to taste.

INSTRUCTIONS
Mix with a fork until consistency of guacamole is even.[49,50]

[49] "Quick and Easy Guacamole: Paleo Leap," Paleo Leap | Paleo diet Recipes & Tips, March 1, 2018, https://paleoleap.com/quick-easy-guacamole/.

[50] M Alvizouri-Muñoz et al., "Effects of Avocado as a Source of Monounsaturated Fatty Acids on Plasma Lipid Levels," Archives of medical research (U.S. National Library of Medicine, 1992), https://www.ncbi.nlm.nih.gov/pubmed/1308699.

40. BASIL

The Why:

Basil is a delicious and powerful herb for healing. This plant should be eaten raw and is easy to grow on your own. Ask any amateur gardener and they'll tell you it'll take over your garden. Loaded with phytochemicals, it's good for digestion (co-enzymes) and highly effective for stomach problems. Pro tip: there are more nutrients in the stems than in the leaves.

The Science:

Clinical studies published in *Nutrition and Cancer* show that basil contains phytochemicals, which can help naturally prevent cancer, including chemical-induced skin, liver, oral and lung cancers. Basil increases antioxidant activity, positively alters gene expressions, induces cancerous-cell apoptosis (death of harmful cells) and stops cancerous tumors from spreading.

In studies using animals, basil extract has shown protection against cancer and mortality while also selectively protecting normal tissue and cells from negative effects of cancer treatments like radiation or chemotherapy. This means that using basil extract can be beneficial as a supplemental cancer treatment even when someone is already undergoing traditional forms of treatments.

The How:

Easy Pesto Recipe:

INGREDIENTS:
2 cups packed fresh basil leaves
2 cloves garlic
1/4 cup pine nuts
2/3 cup extra-virgin olive oil, divided
Kosher salt and freshly ground black pepper, to taste
1/2 cup freshly grated Pecorino cheese

INSTRUCTIONS:
Combine all ingredients in food processor or blender until smooth.[51,52]

[51] "Basil Pesto," Food Network, accessed October 1, 2019,
http://www.foodnetwork.com/recipes/food-network-kitchen/basil-pesto-recipe2.

[52] Manjeshwar Shrinath Baliga et al., "Ocimum Sanctum L (Holy Basil or Tulsi) and
Its Phytochemicals in the Prevention and Treatment of Cancer," Nutrition and cancer
(U.S. National Library of Medicine, 2013),
https://www.ncbi.nlm.nih.gov/pubmed/23682780.

41. BEETS

The Why:

The core principle of healing any disease is in the blood. Beets are nature's blood purifier and liver detoxifier. Their nitrate power has been shown to sharpen your brain and even raise your performance levels if you are into sports.

The Science:

Animal studies have found that beetroot can suppress the development of tumors of the lung and skin. Research has also shown that beetroot extracts can destroy human cancer cells of the prostate and breast. It is thought that betanin, a major compound found in beets, plays a significant role in the fight against cancer cells.

The How:

When beets are cooked, the nitrate content decreases. Moreover, they also lose more than 25% of their folate.

Raw Beet Salad Recipe:

INGREDIENTS

1 to 11/2 pounds beets, preferably small
2 large shallots
Salt and freshly ground black pepper
2 teaspoons Dijon mustard, or to taste
1 tablespoon extra virgin olive oil
2 tablespoons sherry or other good strong vinegar
1 sprig fresh tarragon, minced, if available
1/4 cup chopped parsley leaves

INSTRUCTIONS:

Peel the beets and shallots. Combine them in a food processor and pulse carefully until the beets are shredded; do not purée. (Alternatively, grate the beets by hand and mince the shallots, then combine.) Scrape into a bowl. Toss with the salt, pepper, mustard, oil and vinegar. Taste and adjust the seasoning. Toss in the herbs and serve.[53,54,55]

[53] Govind J. Kapadia et al., "Chemoprevention of Lung and Skin Cancer by Beta Vulgaris (Beet) Root Extract," *Cancer Letters* 100, no. 1-2 (1996): pp. 211-214, https://doi.org/10.1016/0304-3835(95)04087-0.

[54] Govind J. Kapadia et al., "Cytotoxic Effect of the Red Beetroot (Beta Vulgaris L.) Extract Compared to Doxorubicin (Adriamycin) in the Human Prostate (PC-3) and Breast (MCF-7) Cancer Cell Lines," *Anti-Cancer Agents in Medicinal Chemistry* 11, no. 3 (January 2011): pp. 280-284, https://doi.org/10.2174/187152011795347504.

[55] Danielle Omar, Skinny Juices: 101 Juice Recipes for Detox and Weight Loss (Boston, MA: Da Capo Life Long, a member of the Perseus Books Group, 2014).

42. BONE BROTH

The Why:

Bones themselves are rich in vitamins and nutrients, including calcium, magnesium, and phosphorous. The body receives added benefits including natural compounds and collagen from the cartilage, connective tissue and bones. When cooked, collagen becomes gelatin,providing the body with amino acids- the building blocks of proteins.

The Science:

As a 2017 study in the journal *Current Opinion in Clinical Nutrition and Metabolic Care* notes, glutamine helps heal the intestinal barrier in human and animal models. Of the many amino acids available in bone broth glutamine seems very promising in aiding digestion.

This may help with conditions such as leaky gut, which irritates the mucosal lining in the intestines and interferes with the body's ability to digest food.

As a 2017 study in the journal Nutrients says, people with inflammatory bowel disease tend to have lower levels of some amino acids in their bodies. For these people, getting additional amino acids into their diets may help with some symptoms of the condition.

Drinking bone broth daily is a simple way to get anti-inflammatory amino acids into the body.

The How:

Place bones in your stock pot or slow cooker.
Add onion, carrots, celery, salt and peppercorns.
Pour enough water in the pot to cover everything.
Add vinegar and let stand for 30-40 minutes.
Bring to a boil and then reduce to a low simmer for the recommended amount of time:
Chicken bones: 8-24 hours.
Beef bones: 8-72 hours.

Note: Make sure you know the source of your bones. Look for bones from animals that were pastured raised, grass-fed, and without antibiotics.[56,57,58]

[56] Heather Dessinger, "How To Make Bone Broth," MommyPotamus, accessed October 1, 2019, http://www.mommypotamus.com/how-to-make-bone-broth/.

[57] Najate Achamrah, Pierre Déchelotte, and Moïse Coëffier, "Glutamine and the Regulation of Intestinal Permeability: from Bench to Bedside," Current opinion in clinical nutrition and metabolic care (U.S. National Library of Medicine, January 2017), https://www.ncbi.nlm.nih.gov/pubmed/27749689.

[58] Yulan Liu, Xiuying Wang, and Chien-An Andy Hu, "Therapeutic Potential of Amino Acids in Inflammatory Bowel Disease," Nutrients (MDPI, August 23, 2017), https://www.ncbi.nlm.nih.gov/pmc/articles/PMC5622680/.

43. BRUSSELS SPROUTS

The Why:

Brussels sprouts are nature's little ovaries. Like most cruciferous vegetables they contain sulforaphane. Sulforaphane is known to induce colon cells to commit suicide and is great for ovarian disease. Aesthetically, they look like small ovaries.

The Science:

Since the 1980s, consuming high amounts of cruciferous vegetables has been associated with a lower risk of cancer. More recently, researchers have pinpointed the sulfur-containing compounds (namely sulforaphane) that give cruciferous vegetables their bitter bite are also what give them their cancer-fighting power. Diets high in brussels sprouts and other cruciferous vegetables have shown promising results with multiple types of cancers, including melanoma, esophageal, prostate, and pancreatic.

Researchers have discovered that sulforaphane has the power to inhibit the harmful enzyme histone deacetylase (HDAC), known to be involved in the progression of cancer cells. The ability to stop HDAC enzymes could make sulforaphane-containing foods a potentially powerful part of cancer treatment in the future.

Brussels sprouts also contain a high amount of chlorophyll, which can block the carcinogenic effects of heterocyclic amines generated when grilling meats at a high temperature. If you tend to like your grilled foods charred, make sure to pair them with green vegetables to decrease your risk of cancer.

The How:

Preheat oven to 400 degrees F (205 degrees C).
Place trimmed brussels sprouts, olive oil, kosher salt, and pepper in a large resealable plastic bag. Seal tightly, and shake to coat.
Roast in the preheated oven for 30 to 45 minutes, shaking pan every 5 to 7 minutes for even browning.[59]

[59] Corrina et al., "Roasted Brussels Sprouts Recipe," Allrecipes, February 10, 2007, http://allrecipes.com/recipe/67952/roasted-brussels-sprouts/.

44. CARROTS

The Why:

Carrots provide health benefits for our lungs, eyes and digestion. This vitamin A rich food is a foundation for healing through foods. It's one of the foods with the highest levels of special fiber known as pectin. Boiled carrots w/ grass fed butter are a natural remedy for constipation.

The Science:

In a study meant to reveal the therapeutic value of carrots, researchers at the Wolfson Gastrointestinal Laboratory in Edinburgh, Scotland revealed that cholesterol levels drop by an average of 11% percent of seven ounces of raw carrots are eaten per day for three weeks.

A group of Swedish scientists discovered that root vegetables can reduce the chances of having a heart attack. A study conducted at the Mario Negri Institute of Pharmacological Research in Italy found that those who ate more carrots had one-third as high a risk of heart attack as compared with those who ate fewer carrots.[60]

[60] Sari Voutilainen et al., "Carotenoids and Cardiovascular Health," The American journal of clinical nutrition (U.S. National Library of Medicine, June 2006), https://www.ncbi.nlm.nih.gov/pubmed/16762935.

The How:

For 1 to 2 servings use 2 to3 carrots. Cover the pan and cook over medium-low heat for 7 to 8 minutes, until the carrots are just cooked through. Add the butter and saute for another minute, until the water evaporates and the carrots are coated with butter. Remove from heat, toss with dill or parsley. Sprinkle with salt and pepper and serve.[61,62]

61 Meenakshi Nagdeve, "Carrots: Nutrition Facts & Benefits," Organic Facts, September 9, 2019, https://www.organicfacts.net/health-benefits/vegetable/carrots.html.

62 Ina Garten, "Sauteed Carrots," Food Network, accessed October 1, 2019, http://www.foodnetwork.com/recipes/ina-garten/sauteed-carrots-recipe.

45. CAULIFLOWER

The Why:

Antioxidants in Cauliflower

Beta-carotene, beta-cryptoxanthin, caffeic acid, cinnamic acid, ferulic acid, quercetin, rutin, and kaempferol are among cauliflower's key antioxidant phytonutrients. An emphatic addition to this list would be vitamin C since cauliflower is our 10th best source of vitamin C among all 100 whole foods. Like most of its fellow cruciferous vegetables, cauliflower is also a very good source of manganese—a mineral antioxidant that is especially important in oxygen-related metabolism.

The Science:

Several recent studies have shown the cooking of raw cauliflower significantly improves its ability to bind together with bile acids. Since bile acid binding is a well-documented method for helping regulate blood cholesterol levels, these studies point to potential cardiovascular benefits from consumption of cooked cauliflower. The most detailed study that we have seen in this area examined cauliflower that had been steamed for 10 minutes.

The How:

When purchasing cauliflower, look for a clean, creamy white, compact curd in which the bud clusters are not separated. Spotted or dull-colored cauliflower should be avoided, as well as those in which small flowers appear.

Heads that are surrounded by many thick green leaves are better protected and will be fresher. As its size is not related to its quality, choose one that best suits your needs.

Easy Cauliflower Recipe

Preheat the oven to 450 degrees F (220 degrees C).
Grease a large casserole dish.
Place the olive oil and garlic in a large resealable bag.
Add chopped cauliflower, and shake to mix.
Pour into the prepared casserole dish, and season with salt and pepper to taste.
Bake for 25 minutes, stirring halfway through.
Top with Parmesan cheese and parsley, and broil for 3 to 5 minutes, until golden brown.

46. CELERY

The Why:

The health benefits of celery are due to the excellent sources of beneficial enzymes and antioxidants. Celery is loaded with essential minerals and vitamins such as folate, potassium, vitamin B6, vitamin C and vitamin K.

The nutritional value and health benefits of celery have been well studied and it has been used in culinary and folk medicine for centuries. Regular consumption of celery can help protect cardiovascular health. Moreover, the anti-inflammatory and antioxidant properties of celery make it an ideal food for patients with high cholesterol levels and blood pressure, as well as heart disease. Celery also has numerous amazing benefits for skin, liver, eye and cognitive health.

The Science:

Celery contains antioxidants and polysaccharides that are known to act as anti-inflammatories, especially flavonoid and polyphenol antioxidants. These support overall health, especially as you age, by fighting free-radical damage (or oxidative stress) that can lead to inflammation. Inflammation is often a contributing cause of chronic diseases like cancer, heart disease, arthritis and many more.

Researchers have identified over a dozen different types of antioxidants that are responsible for the benefits of celery — these include such phenolic acids as caffeic acid and ferulic acid, plus flavaols like quecetin. This makes celery useful for treating a wide range of conditions that are made worse by inflammation: joint pain (such as from arthritis), gout, kidney and liver infections, skin disorders, irritable bowel syndrome and urinary tract infections, just to name a few.[63]

[63] "Celery, Artichokes Contain Flavonoids That Kill Human Pancreatic Cancer Cells," College of Agricultural, Consumer and Environmental Sciences, accessed October 1, 2019, http://news.aces.illinois.edu/news/celery-artichokes-contain-flavonoids-kill-human-pancreatic-cancer-cells.

http://news.aces.illinois.edu/news/celery-artichokes-contain-flavonoids-kill-human-pancreatic-cancer-cells

The How:

When picking out celery, make sure the stalks seem firm and are not too limber. If the stalks have their leaves attached, look for brightly colored leaves that are not wilting.

Don't wash celery right away after bringing it home because this can cause it go bad more quickly. Store dry celery, wrapped in a paper towel if you'd like, inside the refrigerator for about five to seven days at the most. After this time, celery tends to get limp and its nutrient content starts to decrease. It's also not recommended to freeze celery because it easily wilts and will become mushy once defrosted.

To clean and cut celery, discard the base that's usually firm and white. You can save the leaves and use these in recipes, such as soups or a sauté. Celery leaves are a good source of vitamins and minerals just like the stalks, so don't waste them! Rinse the celery stalks and leaves well to remove any dirt of lingering pesticide spray and then cut the stalks into pieces.[64]

[64] Jillian Levy, "Benefits of Celery Nutrition Facts and Recipes," Dr. Axe, March 7, 2019, https://draxe.com/benefits-of-celery/.

47. COCONUT FLOUR

The Why:

Coconut flour is high in fiber, protein, and healthy fats and is free from wheat and other grains. It is also low in sugar, digestible carbohydrates and calories, and has a low score on the glycemic index.

It is one of the healthier alternatives to white flour when incorporating lower carb, lower glycemic or gluten-free foods in your diet. Due to the many uses as a delicious, gluten-free and beneficial alternative to other flours, coconut flour is growing in popularity as more people discover its many health benefits.

The Science:

Coconut flour is a low glycemic food and does not spike blood sugar levels. This helps maintain a healthy blood sugar level in your body. In fact studies show that consuming products that contain coconut flour can help to lower the overall glycemic impact of the food and to support stable blood sugar levels. This means that coconut flour nutrition has health benefits for people with diabetes and those who are working towards reaching a healthy weight.

The How:

How to Cook with Coconut Flour

Coconut flour can be used in both sweet and savory recipes. It is unsweetened and has a slight smell and taste of coconut, but this easily blends well with other ingredients in recipes and does not overpower other tastes. While it has a light, airy appearance and texture when dried, it becomes pretty dense when cooked or baked with.

You will want to make sure to de-clump the flour first before cooking with it, since it's prone to forming clumps; do this by mixing with a fork to take out any air bubbles or lumpy bits.

Coconut flour is high in fiber with 5 grams per every 2 Tbsp. serving, so it will absorb a lot of water when you cook with it. Compared to other flours, coconut flour is much more of an absorbent "sponge", therefore may dry out certain traditional recipes.

It's best to use coconut flour in combination with other flours or self-rising ingredients like eggs when baking in order to get the best results. Coconut flour can also be used on its own to thicken soups and stews or to coat ingredients in place of breadcrumbs. No matter how you use it, make sure to mix it well before adding it to recipes, and after you've combined it with other ingredients, to ensure you get the best finished product.

48. COCONUT OIL

The Why:

Coconut oil is a staple in every healthy person's diet. It's been reported to aid with digestive disorders and Irritable Bowel Syndrome. Coconut oil is also associated with a beneficial lipid profile in pre-menopausal women in the Philippines.

The Science:

Heart diseases: It is a common misconception that because coconut oil contains a large quantity of saturated fats it is not good for heart health. In reality, it is beneficial for the heart. It contains about 50% lauric acid, which helps to actively prevent various heart problems like high cholesterol levels and high blood pressure. Coconut oil does not lead to an increase in LDL levels, and it reduces the incidence of injury and damage to arteries and therefore helps to prevent atherosclerosis.[65]

[65] Alan B Feranil et al., "Coconut Oil Is Associated with a Beneficial Lipid Profile in Pre-Menopausal Women in the Philippines," Asia Pacific journal of clinical nutrition (U.S. National Library of Medicine, 2011), https://www.ncbi.nlm.nih.gov/pubmed/21669587.

The How:

If you're going to start introducing coconut oil into your diet, go slow and increase the amount over time, otherwise you might experience disaster pants.

Cooking at High Heat (Sauteing and Frying) – Coconut oil is great for cooking at a high heat because of its high smoke point. Many other oils like olive oil can oxidize when heated but because coconut oil is made up of healthy saturated fats it remains stable under high temperatures.[66]

[66] Josh Axe, "77 Coconut Oil Uses," Dr. Axe, May 21, 2018, https://draxe.com/coconut-oil-uses/.

49. COD LIVER OIL

The Why:

Once a standard supplement in traditional European societies, cod liver oil provides fat-soluble vitamins A and D, which Dr. Price (a Canadian dentist known primarily for his theories on the relationship between nutrition, dental health, and physical health) found present in the diet of "primitives" in amounts ten times higher than the typical American diet of his day. Cod liver oil supplements are a must for women and their male partners, to be taken for several months before conception, and for women during pregnancy. Growing children will also benefit greatly from a small daily dose.

Dr. Price always gave cod liver oil with high-vitamin butter oil, extracted by a slow centrifuge from good quality spring or fall butter. He found that cod liver oil on its own was relatively ineffective but combined with butter oil produced excellent results. We now know that butter oil is an excellent source of vitamin K, which is needed to balance vitamins A and D found in cod liver oil.

The Science:

Results from a 2003 study conducted at the University of Oslo in Norway showed that children who were born to mothers who had taken cod liver oil during pregnancy and lactation scored higher on intelligence tests at age four compared with children whose mothers had taken corn oil instead.[67]

[67] Ingrid B Helland et al., "Maternal Supplementation with Very-Long-Chain n-3 Fatty Acids during Pregnancy and Lactation Augments Children's IQ at 4 Years of Age," Pediatrics (U.S. National Library of Medicine, January 2003), https://www.ncbi.nlm.nih.gov/pubmed/12509593.

The How:

Most brands of cod liver oil go through a process that removes all of the natural vitamins. The resulting product contains very low levels of vitamin A and virtually no vitamin D. Some manufacturers add manufactured vitamins A and D to the purified cod liver oil and until recently, one manufacturer added the natural vitamins removed during processing back into the cod liver oil. Fortunately, we now have available in the U.S. a naturally produced, unheated, fermented high-vitamin cod liver oil that is made using a filtering process that retains its natural vitamins.

The high-vitamin fermented cod liver oil is sold as a food and does not contain vitamin levels on the label. However, after numerous tests, the approximate values of A and D have been ascertained at 1900 IU vitamin A per mL and 390 IU vitamin D per mL. Thus 1 teaspoon of high-vitamin fermented cod liver oil contains 9500 IU vitamin A and 1950 IU vitamin D, a ratio of about 5:1.

Based on these values, the dosage for the high-vitamin fermented cod liver oil is provided as follows:

- Children age 3 months to 12 years: 1/2 teaspoon or 2.5 mL, providing 4750 IU vitamin A and 975 IU vitamin D.
- Children over 12 years and adults: 1 teaspoon or 10 capsules, providing 9500 IU vitamin A and 1950 IU vitamin D.
- Pregnant and nursing women: 2 teaspoons or 20 capsules, providing 19,000 IU vitamin A and 3900 IU vitamin D.[68]

[68] Sally Fallon, "Cod Liver Oil Basics and Recommendations," The Weston A. Price Foundation, February 9, 2009, http://www.westonaprice.org/health-topics/cod-liver-oil-basics-and-recommendations/.

50. DARK CHOCOLATE

The Why:

High quality dark chocolate,with a high cocoa content, is actually quite nutritious. It contains a decent amount of soluble fiber and is loaded with minerals.

A 100 gram bar of dark chocolate with 70-85% cocoa contains:

- 11 grams of fiber.
- 67% of the Recommended Daily Allowance (RDA) for Iron.
- 58% of the RDA for Magnesium.
- 89% of the RDA for Copper.
- 98% of the RDA for Manganese.
- It also has plenty of potassium, phosphorus, zinc and selenium.

Of course, 100 grams (3.5 ounces) is a fairly large amount and not something you should consume daily. All these nutrients also come with 600 calories and moderate amounts of sugar.
For this reason, dark chocolate is best consumed in moderation.

The fatty acid profile of cocoa and dark chocolate is excellent. The fats are mostly saturated and monounsaturated, with small amounts of polyunsaturates.

It also contains stimulants like caffeine and theobromine, but is unlikely to keep you awake at night as the amount of caffeine is very small compared to coffee.

The Science:

Dark Chocolate Raises HDL and Protects LDL Against Oxidation

Consuming dark chocolate can improve several important risk factors for heart disease. In a controlled trial, cocoa powder was found to significantly decrease oxidized LDL cholesterol in men. It also increased HDL and lowered total LDL in men with elevated cholesterol. Oxidized LDL means that the LDL ("bad" cholesterol) has reacted with free radicals. This makes the LDL particle itself reactive and capable of damaging other tissues…such as the lining of the arteries in your heart. It makes perfect sense that cocoa lowers oxidized LDL. It contains an abundance of powerful antioxidants are absorbed into the bloodstream and protect lipoproteins against oxidative damage.

Dark chocolate can also reduce insulin resistance, which is another common risk factor for many diseases like heart disease and diabetes.

The How:

You need to choose quality stuff - organic, dark chocolate with 70% or higher cocoa content.

Dark chocolates often contain some sugar, but the amounts are usually small and the darker the chocolate, the less sugar it will contain.

51. EGGS

The Why:

Eggs are considered nature's perfect food - high in quality protein with the right ratios in amino acids, lots of B vitamins, & the "right" kind of cholesterol.

Whole eggs are incredibly nutritious, containing a very large amount of nutrients compared to the calorie load. The nutrients are found in the yolks, while the whites are mostly protein.

The Science:

The main reason people have been warned about eggs is that they're loaded with cholesterol. One large egg contains 212 mg of cholesterol, which is a lot compared to most other foods.

However, just because a food contains cholesterol doesn't mean that it will raise the bad cholesterol in the blood. The liver actually produces cholesterol every single day. The more cholesterol you eat, the less your liver produces. The opposite is also true - if you don't eat enough cholesterol, your liver produces more.

The thing is, many studies show that eggs actually improve your cholesterol profile. Eggs tend to raise HDL (the "good") cholesterol and they tend to change the LDL (the "bad") cholesterol to a large subtype which is not associated with an increased risk of heart disease.

One study discovered that eating three whole eggs per day reduced insulin resistance, raised HDL and increased the size of LDL particles in men and women with metabolic syndrome.

Multiple studies have examined the effects of egg consumption on the risk of cardiovascular disease and found no association between the two.

However, some studies do show an increased risk of cardiovascular disease in diabetic patients. This needs further research and probably does not apply on a low-carb diet, which can in many cases reverse type II diabetes.

The How:

Not All Eggs Are The Same.

It's important to keep in mind that not all eggs are created equal.

Hens are often raised in factories, caged and fed grain-based feed that alters the final nutrient composition of the eggs. It is best to buy Omega-3 enriched or pastured eggs as they are more nutritious and better for you.[69,70]

[69] Christopher N Blesso et al., "Whole Egg Consumption Improves Lipoprotein Profiles and Insulin Sensitivity to a Greater Extent than Yolk-Free Egg Substitute in Individuals with Metabolic Syndrome," Metabolism: clinical and experimental (U.S. National Library of Medicine, March 2013), https://www.ncbi.nlm.nih.gov/pubmed/23021013.

[70] Maria L Fernandez, "Rethinking Dietary Cholesterol," Current opinion in clinical nutrition and metabolic care (U.S. National Library of Medicine, March 2012), https://www.ncbi.nlm.nih.gov/pubmed/22037012.

52. GARLIC

The Why:

There have been entire books dedicated to the health and healing benefits of garlic. I.e. *Garlic: Nature's Natural Companion*. Garlic is a prebiotic food that helps get your probiotics ready for your system. Raw garlic is also known to remove candida (bad yeast bacteria) from your system. Using plenty of cooked and raw garlic in your cooking is not only good for you, it. makes your food taste delicious.

The Science:

The active compounds in garlic can reduce blood pressure. Cardiovascular diseases like heart attacks and strokes are the world's biggest killers. High blood pressure, or hypertension, is one of the most important drivers of these diseases. Studies have found garlic supplementation to have a significant impact on reducing blood pressure in people with high blood pressure.

In one study, aged garlic extract at doses of 600-1,500 mg was just as effective as the drug Atenolol at reducing blood pressure over a 24 week period. Supplement doses must be fairly high to have these desired effects. The amount of allicin (chemical organosulfur compound) needed is equivalent to about four cloves of garlic per day.

The How:

- Get a garlic bulb and separate a clove, one of the small, wedge-shaped pieces that make up the entire "head" of garlic.
- Place the clove on a chopping board.
- Peel away the skin and waste with your hands.
- Use the peeled clove, either chopped or full.[71,72]

[71] Rizwan Ashraf et al., "Effects of Allium Sativum (Garlic) on Systolic and Diastolic Blood Pressure in Patients with Essential Hypertension," Pakistan journal of pharmaceutical sciences (U.S. National Library of Medicine, September 2013), https://www.ncbi.nlm.nih.gov/pubmed/24035939.

[72] Person and wikiHow, "How to Peel a Garlic Clove," wikiHow (wikiHow, May 2, 2019), http://www.wikihow.com/Peel-a-Garlic-Clove.

53. GHEE

The Why:

Ghee has been used for thousands of years dating back to 2000 BC. It is truly an "ancient" health food. Ghee quickly was integrated into the diet, ceremonial practice and Ayurvedic healing practices and today its health benefits (Vitamins. A, D E) are being discovered by modern science. It's believed to promote both mental and physical purification through its ability to cleanse and support wellness. Ghee benefits the body both inside and out, and is actually used topically to treat burns and rashes as well as to moisturize the skin and scalp. Much like coconut oil, it's a multi-use fat that is healthy in many ways!

The Science:

Ghee contains butyrate, an essential short-chain fatty acid, that acts as a detoxifier and improves colon health. It's been shown to support healthy insulin levels, is an anti-inflammatory, and may be helpful for individuals suffering from IBS, Crohn's disease and ulcerative colitis.

A recent study found that "butyrate can prevent and treat diet-induced insulin resistance in mouse." Researchers agree that more study needs to be conducted to further explore how butyrate affects insulin levels in humans.[73]

The How:

Anyone can make ghee. When made with grass-fed butter, the home process retains more nutrients than ghee made in a centrifuge in commercial products. Here is what you need to get started:

---

[73] Zhanguo Gao et al., "Butyrate Improves Insulin Sensitivity and Increases Energy Expenditure in Mice," Diabetes (American Diabetes Association, July 1, 2009), http://diabetes.diabetesjournals.org/content/58/7/1509.long.

INGREDIENTS/MATERIALS:

1 pound of grass-fed unsalted butter
Deep, wide-bottomed skilled
Wooden spoon or heat-resistant spatula
Cheesecloth
Mesh skimmer
Mesh strainer
Glass jar

INSTRUCTIONS:

Place one pound of butter into a deep skillet over medium-low heat and watch it melt. Do not try to rush this step.The key here is to melt the butter slowly. As the butter begins to bubble, it will spatter a bit. Stir with a long-handled spoon and maintain a simmer.

Continue to simmer, stirring occasionally, for 20 to30 minutes until the milk proteins have separated from the gold liquid. There will be white foam on the top, and some bits of milk fats on the bottom of the pan. Gently skim the foam off with the mesh skimmer and discard. You may have another "foam up" stage, and this is good. Skim and discard once again. Now, the milk fats on the bottom of the pan will continue to brown. Again, this is a good thing – this is where the distinctive nutty flavor comes from.

Continue to simmer until the milk fats are golden brown, but not burnt. Keep a watchful eye because at this stage, the ghee can quickly burn. Remove from heat and allow to cool to room temperature. Place several layers of cheesecloth in the mesh strainer (or use nut milk bags) and slowly pour the butter into the jar. The result? A beautiful golden clarified butter that is liquid gold.

While it will firm up a bit at room temperature, keep in the refrigerator if you desire a spreadable ghee. Ghee will remain fresh at room temperature for several weeks, when sealed properly. It can last months in the refrigerator. Because fats tend to absorb other flavors, it's essential that ghee is kept properly sealed whether in the refrigerator or on the counter.

54. GINGER

The Why:

Ginger is nature's master anti-inflammation herb. This root has phytochemicals structurally similar to the COX2 inhibitors found in Advil & Aleve.

The Chinese and Indians have used ginger tonics to treat ailments for more than 4,700 years, and during the Roman Empire trade around the coming of Christ it was a priceless commodity because of its medicinal properties.

The Science:

Gingerol is what makes ginger so good for us. Of the 115 different chemical components found in ginger root, the therapeutic benefits come from gingerols, the oily resin from the root that acts as a highly potent antioxidant and anti-inflammatory agent. These bioactive ingredients, especially gingerol, have been thoroughly evaluated clinically, and the research backs up why you should use ginger on a regular basis.

The Journal of Microbiology and Antimicrobials published a study in 2011 that tested just how effective ginger is in enhancing immune function. Comparing the ability of ginger to kill Staphylococcus aureus and Streptococcus pyogenes *(infectious bacteria)* with conventional antibiotics, Nigerian researchers discovered that the natural solution won every time!

The drugs — chloramphenicol, ampicillin and tetracycline — just couldn't stand up to the antibacterial prowess of the ginger extract. This is important because these two bacteria are extremely common in hospitals and oftentimes cause complications to an already immune-compromised patient.

The How:

Look for large, plump pieces of ginger root that are moist and heavy for their size. This will give you more ginger to work with. Also look for pieces of ginger root that are straight and rectangular in shape, with as few bumps and knobs as possible. This will make them easier to peel and prepare. Ginger root can be frozen, unpeeled, for up to 6 months, so do not be afraid to buy more than you need for your current recipe.

55. GO BOOZE FREE

The Why:

Having fun without the aid of alcohol is a not a skill everyone has. Those that have learned this skill can interact with a buzzed crowd, get 'high' off the energy of the conversations, have great time and wake up without the consequences. Like any skills it takes practice and persistence to master.

The Science:

Alcohol has a sneaky way of increasing your daily calorie intake without you realizing it. One margarita may contain 300 calories or more—mostly from sugar. (A delicious piña colada might have 450 calories!) One study found men consume an additional 433 calories on those days they drink a "moderate" amount of alcohol. For women, it's 300 calories. Cut those from your diet—and don't replace them with desserts—and you'll start to lose weight without much effort.[74]

---

[74] Breslow, Rosalind A., and Barbara A., "Drinking Patterns and Body Mass Index in Never Smokers: National Health Interview Survey, 1997–2001," OUP Academic (Oxford University Press, February 15, 2005), http://aje.oxfordjournals.org/content/161/4/368.full.

The How:

Here are 5 tips for giving up booze.

1. If you are looking for support, tell a friend who already does not drink a lot.
2. Be ready to learn about the quality and depth of your friendships. Telling your drinking buddy that you are not drinking will answer this question. Is there more to our friendship than sharing a drink?
3. Be ready to learn about yourself. You'll start to answer this question. "Am I only capable of having fun with I'm drinking?"
4. When out in a bar, order a club soda and lime, and pretend there is alcohol in it. You'll be surprised how 'drunk' you think you are.
5. Don't tell anyone you're not drinking. It'll derail into a therapy session about their drinking justifications. Simply have a good time, enjoy your friends, and a free bar tab.[75]

[75] Paul, "10 Tips to Stop Drinking Alcohol," Stop Drinking Alcohol, July 28, 2016, http://stopdrinkingalcohol.com/10-tips-stop-drinking-alcohol/.

56. GOJI BERRIES

The Why:

Goji berries have been used in traditional Chinese medicine for more than 2,000 years.

All dark blue or red berries, including goji berries, contain high levels of antioxidants, which may help protect the body against damage from free radicals.

What's unique about goji berries is that they contain specific antioxidants called Lycium barbarum polysaccharides, which are thought to provide a variety of impressive health benefits.

In addition, goji berries provide 11 essential amino acids — more than other common berries.

The Science:

One study in healthy elderly men and women found that taking a milk-based goji berry drink daily for 90 days increased levels of the antioxidant zeaxanthin by 26%, and increased overall antioxidant capacity by 57%.

The How:

Goji berries are typically found in the bulk section of your local health food store.

Store dried goji berries in a cool, dark place (your pantry is just fine). They'll keep for at least a year, though brands that package the berries with added preservatives may advertise a longer shelf life. Make sure to keep the dried berries away from moisture to prevent them from clumping.[76]

[76] Peter Bucheli et al., "Goji Berry Effects on Macular Characteristics and Plasma Antioxidant Levels," Optometry and vision science: official publication of the American Academy of Optometry (U.S. National Library of Medicine, February 2011), https://www.ncbi.nlm.nih.gov/pubmed/21169874.

57. GRASS-FED BUTTER

The Why:

One of the many beneficial vitamins we get from butter is vitamin A, which has a wide range of functions for our bodies. Grass-fed butter has even more vitamin A than regular butter thanks to the cow's healthier grass-centric diet. Compared to standard butter, grass-fed butter can have 3% or more vitamin A per tablespoon. This might not sound like a lot, but over the course of a day and a lifetime, that added vitamin A can really add up.

Vitamin A plays a crucial role in the formation and maintenance of not only your teeth, skeletal and soft tissue, but also your mucus membranes and skin. Vitamin A is also needed to maintain good vision, especially at night or other low-light situations. Vitamin A is essential to proper endocrine system function as well, along with reproduction and breastfeeding.

The Science:

A heart study published in the journal Epidemiology looked at the effects of butter and margarine on cardiovascular disease. Margarine consumption increased the risk of coronary heart disease, while butter intake was not at all associated with coronary heart disease occurrence.

Another 16-year prospective study published in the European Journal of Clinical Nutrition in 2010 evaluated whether the intake of dairy products or related nutrients is linked with mortality due to cardiovascular disease (CVD). The researchers found that overall the intake of dairy products was not associated with dying from CVD or cancer. In comparison to the study subjects with the lowest full-fat intake of dairy products, the participants with the highest intake (median intake was 339 grams per day) actually had reduced death rate due to CVD after adjustment for calcium intake and other variables.

The How:

The ideal butter is:

- From grass-fed cows.
- Organic.
- Unsalted or sea-salted (unfortunately, many organic butters often use inferior salt rather than sea salt).
- Made from raw milk or fermented milk.[77,78,79]

[77] M W Gillman et al., "Margarine Intake and Subsequent Coronary Heart Disease in Men," Epidemiology (Cambridge, Mass.) (U.S. National Library of Medicine, March 1997), https://www.ncbi.nlm.nih.gov/pubmed/9229205.

[78] M Bonthuis et al., "Dairy Consumption and Patterns of Mortality of Australian Adults," Nature News (Nature Publishing Group, April 7, 2010), https://www.nature.com/articles/ejcn201045.

[79] Annie Price, "Grass-Fed Butter Nutrition Benefits & More," Dr. Axe, January 2, 2017, https://draxe.com/grass-fed-butter-nutrition/.

58. GRASS-FED CALVES LIVER

The Why:

Grass-fed calves liver is one of the most nutrient dense meats out there. It's rich in vitamin B12 (brain function) & iron (red blood cells).

The Science:

Most animal foods contain some amount of vitamin B12, but by far, the best source is liver which should be eaten at least once a week. Many disorders of the nervous system result from vitamin B12 deficiency causing a myriad of illnesses and behaviors. So if you are experiencing vague symptoms (related to a less than optimal functioning brain and nervous system) such as difficulty in thinking and remembering, panic attacks, weakness, loss of balance, numbness in the hands and feet, or agitated depression, make sure that your source of vitamin B12 is from healthy animal products, especially a premium source of liver. Vitamin B12 is only well absorbed from animal sources, with liver being the most concentrated source.

The How:

Calf Liver Recipe:
Ingredients

- 2 pounds sliced beef liver.
- 1 ½ cup of organic whole milk
- 2 cup all purpose flour
- 1/2 teaspoon sea salt
- 1/2 teaspoon pepper
- ½ cup tablespoons clarified butter

1. Gently rinse liver slices under cold water, and place in a medium bowl. Pour in enough milk to cover. Let stand while preparing onions. (I like to soak up to an hour or two - whatever you have time for.) This step is SO important in taking the bitter taste of the liver out.

2. Melt 2 tablespoons of butter in a large skillet over medium heat. Separate onion rings, and saute them in butter until soft. Remove onions, and melt remaining butter in the skillet. Season the flour with salt and pepper, and put it in a shallow dish or on a plate. Drain milk from liver, and coat slices in the flour mixture.

3. When the butter has melted, turn the heat up to medium-high, and place the coated liver slices in the pan. Cook until nice and brown on the bottom. Turn, and cook on the other side until browned. Add onions, and reduce heat to medium. Cook a bit longer to taste. Our family prefers the liver to just barely retain a pinkness on the inside when you cut to check. Enjoy!

Pro tip: if you can't take the taste mix, cooked liver with other meats or cut into pill like servings.[80]

[80] Alexandra Rowles, "Why Liver Is a Nutrient-Dense Superfood," Healthline, June 7, 2017, https://www.healthline.com/nutrition/why-liver-is-a-superfood#section1.

59. GRASS-FED CHEESE

The Why:

100% grass-fed cheese comes from cows that have grazed in pasture year-round rather than being fed a processed diet for much of their life. Grass feeding improves the quality of the cheese and results in cheese that is richer in omega-3 fats, vitamin E, and CLA (a beneficial fatty acid named "conjugated linoleic acid".)

The Science:

Research on food and type 2 diabetes has typically focused on foods that are rich in both protein and fiber, with less attention paid to animal foods like cheese that are rich in protein but don't contain fiber. However, a recent study from Denmark has shown better regulation of blood sugar levels following moderate intake of cheese (a little less than one ounce per day). In fact, consumption not only of cheese, but also of fermented dairy foods in general (like yogurt), were associated with some blood sugar benefits. The researchers suggested that the presence of two fat-soluble vitamins — vitamins K and D— in cheese was as a possible reason for these benefits. Both vitamins have been shown to play a role in blood sugar regulation. Due to the use of vitamin K-synthesizing bacteria as a way to start the cheese fermentation process, vitamin K is present in most cheeses in the form of menaquinone. Vitamin D is present in cheese as a naturally occurring nutrient in cow's milk or as a vitamin added during milk fortification. The calcium-rich nature of cheese may also play a role in beneficial regulation of blood sugar since calcium deficiency—especially in combination with vitamin D deficiency—is a known risk factor for blood sugar problems.

The How:

Stick with organic

Organic standards help lower risk of contaminated feed and organic cheese usually has higher nutrient quality. However, remember that organic by itself does not guarantee a natural lifestyle for the dairy cows.

Ask for 100% grass-fed

Go beyond organic by asking for 100% grass-fed. Don't get sidetracked by the confusing array of labeling terms like "natural" or "pasture-raised." Labeling laws allow products to display these terms even if dairy cows spend little or no time outdoors in a pasture setting. Unfortunately, even the term "grass-fed" is not sufficient since grass-fed dairy cows may have spent a relatively small amount of time grass feeding. The standard to look for on the label is "100% grass-fed." Talk to your grocer or the dairy cow farmer and find out how the animals were actually raised.

Consider local farms

Organic, 100% grass-fed cheese may be available from local farms with small flocks, which provide a natural lifestyle for their dairy cows. Two websites that can help you find small local farms in your area are www.localharvest.org and www.eatwild.com. Both sites are searchable by zip code.

60. GREEN TEA

The Why:

Nothing beats a warm cup of green tea! This aromatic beverage is a rich source of antioxidants, boasting the ability to reduce cholesterol and lower blood pressure. A cup on a daily basis is a surefire way to regulate blood sugar levels and even boost your immunity and metabolism. To top it off, green tea can help ease stress and promote a sense of well-being.

Drinking tea is a great warming agent for the body. Due to its antioxidants and phytochemicals its been shown to help with cardiovascular disease and cancer prevention as an immune system booster.

The Science:

Compared to other types of tea, green tea has a noteworthy level of antioxidant activity. It contains higher levels of epigallocatechin gallate (EGCG), a polyphenol that has potent cancer-fighting abilities. This component is actually lost in the fermentation process used to make black tea. Researchers even found that it helps battle the big C by inducing death of cancer cells. During the study, they compared the activity of different phenolic acids along with the flavonoids in green tea. The conclusion? Epigallocatechin gallate was most effective in its antiproliferative action against cancerous cells. So, if you're torn between black or green tea, go for green tea for an antioxidant boost.

The How:

Look for antioxidant content.

The main antioxidant found in green tea, epigallocatechin gallate (EGCG) varies in amount from brand to brand. Consumerlabs.com recently tested 24 brands of green tea to find out their EGCG content and found that Lipton Green Tea, Teavana Gyokuro Imperial Green Tea, and Harney & Sons Organic Green Tea had the most antioxidants.

Choose loose leaf tea.

The same Consumerlabs.com study also found that tea that came from loose leaves tended to be the most potent source of EGCG.

Avoid added sugars.

Many iced green tea varieties add sugar to their brew. This adds calories in a place where it's totally unnecessary. If you want to add a bit of honey to hot tea, that's just fine, but don't let sugar take over your brew.

Make sure it's fresh.

Green tea doesn't stay fresh for long periods of time. It has a shelf life of about six months and then its freshness begins to diminish. You can extend its shelf life by refrigerating it for a few extra months.

Brew your tea correctly.

Generally, one teaspoon of loose green tea is enough for one 8 ounce cup. I usually add it to a French press with scalding water and brew for 2 to 3 minutes.

Choose first harvest tea.

Green tea quality is separated into harvests, the first harvest being the best. The highest quality tea leaves are picked the earliest in the year between March and April. Kabusecha green tea, for example, comes from the first harvest. It has a grassy aroma and it tastes great.

Choose organic green tea.

Make sure your green tea is organic so you can avoid contamination with pesticides and chemicals. Make sure you're getting simple, organic green tea leaves and nothing else.[81,82,83]

[81] Sara Novak, "Green Tea Benefits: 7 Tips For Choosing The Best Brew," Organic Authority, September 10, 2014, http://www.organicauthority.com/green-tea-benefits-7-tips-for-choosing-the-best-brew/.

[82] Tsung O. Cheng, "All Teas Are Not Created Equal: The Chinese Green Tea and Cardiovascular Health," International Journal of Cardiology 108, no. 3 (2006): pp. 301-308, https://doi.org/10.1016/j.ijcard.2005.05.038.

[83] Guang-Jian Du et al., "Epigallocatechin Gallate (EGCG) Is the Most Effective Cancer Chemopreventive Polyphenol in Green Tea," Nutrients 4, no. 11 (August 2012): pp. 1679-1691, https://doi.org/10.3390/nu4111679.

61. HONEY

The Why:

Honey is a real food that has been accessible to humans throughout evolutionary history and can still be obtained in its natural form.

Unrefined honey contains an abundance of various antioxidants that can have major implications for health. Generally speaking, antioxidants in the diet are associated with improved health and lower risk of disease.

The Science:

One study reported a 43.3% success rate with honey as a wound treatment. In another study, topical honey healed a whopping 97% of patients being treated for their diabetic ulcers .

Researchers believe that its healing powers come from its antibacterial and anti-inflammatory effects, as well as its ability to nourish the surrounding tissue.

What's more, it can help treat other skin conditions, including psoriasis, hemorrhoids and herpes lesions.

The How:

Honey is a delicious, healthier alternative to refined sugar.

Make sure to choose a high-quality brand, as some of the lower-quality ones may be adulterated with syrup.

Keep in mind that honey should only be consumed in moderation, as it is still high in calories and sugar.

The benefits of honey are most pronounced when it is replacing another unhealthier sweetener.

At the end of the day, honey is simply a "less bad" sweetener than sugar and high-fructose corn syrup.[84,85]

[84] A M Moghazy et al., "The Clinical and Cost Effectiveness of Bee Honey Dressing in the Treatment of Diabetic Foot Ulcers," Diabetes research and clinical practice (U.S. National Library of Medicine, September 2010), https://www.ncbi.nlm.nih.gov/pubmed/20646771.

[85] Alexandros V Kamaratos et al., "Manuka Honey-Impregnated Dressings in the Treatment of Neuropathic Diabetic Foot Ulcers," International wound journal (U.S. National Library of Medicine, June 2014), https://www.ncbi.nlm.nih.gov/pubmed/22985336.

62. KEFIR

The Why:

Kefir contains many compounds and nutrients, like biotin and folate, that help kick your immune system into gear and protect your cells. It has a large amounts of probiotics, the special forces of the microbial world. One in particular that's specific to kefir alone is called Lactobacillus Kefiri, and it helps defend against harmful bacteria like salmonella and E. Coli. This bacterial strain, along with the various others handfuls, helps modulate the immune system and inhibit many predatory bacteria growth.

Kefir also contains another powerful compound found only in this probiotic drink, an insoluble polysaccharide called kefiran that's been shown to be antimicrobial and help to fight against candida. Kefiran has also shown the ability to lower cholesterol and blood pressure.

The Science:

Kefir benefits in the fight against cancer are due to its large anti-carcinogenic role inside the body. It can slow the growth of early tumors and their enzymatic conversions from non-carcinogenic to carcinogenic. One in-vitro test conducted by the School of Dietetics and Human Nutrition at the Macdonald Campus of McGill University in Canada showed that kefir reduced breast cancer cells by 56% (as opposed to yogurt strains that reduced cells by 14%) in animal studies.

The How:

If you want to make your own kefir, you can buy powder starters. These powders typically contain roughly seven to nine strains of bacteria and are good for people who don't want to have a continuous batch of kefir grains to maintain. Unlike packets or store-bought kefir, kefir grains are self-sustainable since they actually grow and make new grains at a rate of 10% to 15% each time they're fed. Genuine kefir grains themselves carry over 40 strains of probiotics and must be transferred immediately from batch to batch to remain active and alive. Another unique positive to making your own kefir is homemade kefir is often carbonated as opposed to the packaged kind.

You may also use water kefir as a substitute for traditional milk kefir if you're a vegan. Water kefir uses crystal or salt-like grains instead of the white, cloudy type and feeds off of sugar instead of lactose. It provides most, if not all, of the same kefir benefits but has a slightly different, fizzy taste and mouthfeel. It's clear or colored by juice as opposed to milky in appearance as well, and it's in the family of kombucha.

It's important if you're buying grains online for both milk and water kefir to buy from a reputable dealer who packages them fresh and has not previously dehydrated the grains. If you purchase the grains, they should be shipped overnight or express.

If you want to take a break from your kefir making, you may also store the grains in the refrigerator or a cool place, covered with sugar water or fresh milk. Change out the milk every couple of weeks. It's important not to squeeze out the grains or wash them with soap or detergent. Transfer and store them using non-metallic surfaces, utensils and containers. You may also rinse off the grains if they begin to go bad, but only use cold spring water. If you're considering storing them, please note you will have to spend a few days "waking them" back up with a process of sugar feedings.[86,87]

[86] Emma Christensen, "How To Make Milk Kefir," Kitchn (Apartment Therapy, LLC., June 9, 2019), http://www.thekitchn.com/how-to-make-milk-kefir-cooking-lessons-from-the-kitchn-202022.

[87] Marina L Ritchie and Tamara N Romanuk, "A Meta-Analysis of Probiotic Efficacy for Gastrointestinal Diseases," PloS one (Public Library of Science, 2012), https://www.ncbi.nlm.nih.gov/pubmed/22529959.

63. KIMCHI

The Why:

Kimchi is a natural source of probiotics. Eating just a forkful (or chopstick) full will increase the good guys in your immune system. Many people find that consuming fermented foods helps kill their sugar addiction, improves digestion and helps with appetite regulation. If weight loss is your primary goal, kimchi is very low in calories but high in nutrients and satiating fiber.

The Science:

Kimchi is chock-full of anti-inflammatory foods and spices that are known to be cancer-fighting foods. They promote overall better health and longevity and slow down oxidative stress. For example, different color varieties of cabbage can contribute a range of important antioxidant and anti-inflammatory compounds to your diet. Garlic, ginger, radishes, red pepper and scallions are also high in antioxidant properties that help lower inflammation. Anti-inflammatory foods are important for preventing chronic diseases associated to oxidative stress, such as cancer, cognitive disorders and coronary artery diseases.

Research suggests that the compound capsaicin, which is contained in the red hot pepper powder, helps reduce the chance of developing lung cancer. Several population studies demonstrate an association between an increased intake of garlic and reduced risk of certain cancers, including cancers of the stomach, colon, esophagus, pancreas and breast. In addition, the indole-3-carbinol contained in Chinese cabbage has been linked to decreased gut inflammation and chance of colon cancer.

The How:

You can buy jarred kimchi in health food stores, specialty Asian grocery stores and some major chain grocery stores.

There are typically three kimchi products you can choose from in stores:

1. Freshly-packed items of salad-type kimchi called Geotjeori–fresh kimchi, seasoned, without fermentation
2. Refrigerated items of fermented kimchi
3. Fermented, pasteurized items of shelf-stable kimchi.

I recommend choosing the second option, which is most health-boosting. Opt for fermented but not pasteurized kimchi.

64. KOMBUCHA

The Why:

Known as the "Immortal Health Elixir" by the Chinese and originating in the Far East around 2,000 years ago, kombucha is a beverage with tremendous health benefits extending to your heart, your brain and especially your gut. This fermented tea is tasty, filled with probiotics, and supports digestion. It is also a good alternative for people weaning themselves off soda.

The Science:

The research is still out on the specific way Kombucha affects digestion, but we do know that it contains probiotics, enzymes and beneficial acids that have been researched for their health benefits.

Harvard Medical School explains that a healthy gut will have 100 trillion+ microorganisms from 500 different identified species. In this sense, we truly are more bacterial than human. There is a lot of emerging research on the dangers of an overly sanitary environment and how overuse of antibiotics and antibacterial soaps and products is literally changing the structure of our gut.

Drinks like Kombucha, Water Kefir, Milk Kefir, and fermented foods like sauerkraut contain billions of the beneficial bacteria, enzymes and acids that help keep the gut in balance.

The How:

You need:

- 1 large glass or metal jar or bowl with a wide opening — Avoid using a plastic jar or bowl because the chemicals in the plastic can leach into the kombucha during the fermentation period.

Ceramic pots might leach into the kombucha once the acid comes into contact with the ceramic glaze. Look for a big metal or glass jug/jar/bowl, and make sure the opening is wide enough to allow a lot of oxygen to reach the kombucha while it ferments.

- 1 large piece of cloth or a dish towel — Secure this material around the opening of the jar with a rubber band. Do not use a cheesecloth, as it allows particles to pass through. You can even try using an old thin cotton T-shirt or some simple cotton fabric from any textile store.

- 1 SCOBY disk — You can find a SCOBY disk in health food stores or online for relatively inexpensive amounts. A SCOBY disk can be vacuum-sealed in a small pouch and shipped directly to your house for only a few dollars, while still preserving all of the active yeast ingredients.

- 8 cups of water — use filtered water, if possible, but tap water is also a viable option. Some prefer using distilled water, which contains less contaminants or metals than tap water. Distilled water is inexpensive (around 88 cents a gallon) and can be found at most large drug or convenience stores.

- ½ cup organic cane sugar or raw honey — Yes, this is one of the few times I'll tell you to use real sugar! Most of it is actually "eaten" by the yeast during the fermentation process, so there is very little sugar left in the recipe by the time you consume it. It is important to use only organic cane sugar. There are reports of successful kombucha fermentation using raw honey, but most sources recommend cane sugar only.

- 4 organic tea bags — Traditionally, kombucha is made from black tea, but you can also try green tea to see which you prefer.

- 1 cup of pre-made kombucha — You need to purchase your first batch or get a cup from a friend who has recently made homemade kombucha. For future batches, just keep a cup on hand for the next time. Be sure to purchase only organic, unpasteurized kombucha. Pasteurized varieties do not contain the appropriate live cultures you need.

Directions:

- Bring your water to boil in a big pot on the stovetop. Once boiling, remove from heat and add your teabags and sugar, stirring until the sugar dissolves.
- Allow the pot to sit and the tea to steep for about 15 minutes, then remove and discard tea bags.
- Let the mixture cool down to room temperature (which usually takes about one hour). Once it's cool, add your tea mixture to your big jar/bowl. Drop in your SCOBY disk and 1 cup of pre-made kombucha.
- Cover your jar/bowl with your cloth or thin kitchen towel and try to keep the cloth in place by using a rubber band or some sort of tie. You want the cloth to cover the wide opening of the jar and stay in place but be thin enough to allow air to pass through.
- Allow the kombucha to sit for 7–10 days, depending on the flavor you're looking for. Less time produces a weaker kombucha that tastes less sour, while a longer sitting time makes the kombucha ferment even longer and develop more taste. Some people report fermenting kombucha for up to a month before bottling with great results, so taste test the batch every couple of days to see if it's reached the right taste and level of carbonation for you.[88]

[88] "Cultures For Health," Cultures for Health, January 25, 2019, http://www.culturesforhealth.com/learn/kombucha/how-to-make-kombucha/.

65. LEAFY GREENS

The Why:

Leafy Greens are nature's multi-vitamin. They have almost all the nutrients our body needs. This is why the salad's base vegetable is a leafy green. The more varied the leafy green the more vitamins.

The Science:

Studies have identified a gene, connexin 43, whose expression is upregulated by chemopreventive carotenoids and which allows direct intercellular gap junctional communication. In many human tumors gap junctional communication is deficient and its up-regulation is associated with decreased proliferation. Hence, the cancer-preventive properties of carotenoids are partly explained by their impact on gene regulation.[89]

[89] Li-Xin Zhang, Robert V. Cooney, and John S. Bertram, "Carotenoids Up-Regulate Connexin43 Gene Expression Independent of Their Provitamin A or Antioxidant Properties," Cancer Research (American Association for Cancer Research, October 15, 1992), http://cancerres.aacrjournals.org/content/52/20/5707.

The How:

Green, leafy vegetables provide a great variety of colors from the bluish-green of kale to the bright kelly green of spinach. Leafy greens run the whole gamut of flavors, from sweet to bitter, from peppery to earthy. Young plants generally have small, tender leaves and a mild flavor. Many mature plants have tougher leaves and stronger flavors. Collards, Swiss chard, bok choy, and spinach provide a mild flavor while arugula, mizuna and mustard greens provide a peppery flavor. Bok choy is best known for use in stir-fries, since it remains crisp even when cooked to a tender stage. When choosing greens, look for crisp leaves that have a fresh vibrant green color. Yellowing is a sign of age and indicates that the greens may have an off flavor. Salad greens provide a whole range of important nutrients and phytochemicals to keep us healthy. [90]

[90] Neha and Susan George, "Vegetarian Nutrition," Vegetarian Nutrition, January 1, 1966, https://vegetarian-nutrition.info/green-leafy-vegetables/.

66. LEMONS

The Why:

In addition to their unique phytonutrient properties, lemons are an excellent source of vitamin C, one of the most important antioxidants in nature. Vitamin C is one of the main antioxidants found in food and the primary water-soluble antioxidant in the body. Vitamin C travels through the body neutralizing any free radicals it comes into contact with in the aqueous environments in the body both inside and outside cells. Free radicals can interact with the healthy cells of the body, damaging them and their membranes, and also cause a lot of inflammation, or painful swelling, in the body. This is one of the reasons that vitamin C has been shown to be helpful for reducing some of the symptoms of osteoarthritis and rheumatoid arthritis.

The Science:

Lemons have the potential of protection against rheumatoid arthritis. While one study suggests that high doses of supplemental vitamin C makes osteoarthritis, a type of degenerative arthritis that occurs with aging, worse in laboratory animals, another indicates that vitamin C-rich foods, such as lemons, provide humans with protection against inflammatory polyarthritis, a form of rheumatoid arthritis involving two or more joints.

The findings, presented in the Annals of the Rheumatic Diseases were drawn from a study of more than 20,000 subjects who kept diet diaries and were arthritis-free when the study began, and focused on subjects who developed inflammatory polyarthritis and similar subjects who remained arthritis-free during the follow-up period. Subjects who consumed the lowest amounts of vitamin C-rich foods were more than three times more likely to develop arthritis than those who consumed the highest amounts.

The How:

One of the tricks to finding a good quality lemon is to find one that is rather thin-skinned. Lemons with thicker peels will have less flesh and therefore be less juicy. Choose lemons that are heavy for their size and that feature peels that have a finely grained texture. They should be fully yellow in color as those that have green tinges have not fully ripened and will be more acidic. Signs of overmature fruit include wrinkling, soft or hard patches and dull coloring. Fresh lemons are available all year round.

67. MUSHROOMS

The Why:

Fun with fungi. Out of the 14,000 species of mushroom, a type of fungi, only 3,000 are edible. 700 of these mushroom species are said to have medicinal properties.

Mushrooms also have the natural ability to fight dangerous bacteria and viruses. In fact, mushrooms need to have strong antibacterial and antifungal compounds just to survive in their own natural environment, which is why it's not surprising that these beneficial compounds can be isolated from many mushrooms and used to protect human cells.

The Science:

According to a 2005 report published in the Journal of Evidence-Based Complementary and Alternative Medicine, mushrooms contain "compounds and complex substances with antimicrobial, antiviral, antitumor, antiallergic, immunomodulating, anti-inflammatory, antiatherogenic, hypoglycemic, and hepatoprotective activities."

This means mushrooms can enhance almost every system in the body and protect you from numerous diseases since they're associated with lowered inflammation, which is the root of most diseases. Mushrooms also help alkalize the body, which is associated with improved immunity. A balanced pH level is crucial to health because, as some experts say, "disease cannot grow in an alkaline environment."

Mushrooms are even shown to have special fighting abilities against deadly multi-resistant bacterial strains and microorganisms responsible for gut and skin problems. In fact, some substances present in common antibiotics given to people when they're sick, including penicillin, streptomycin and tetracycline are derived from mushroom fungal extracts.

The How:

Mushroom Recipe

Heat olive oil and butter in a large saucepan over medium heat. Cook and stir mushrooms, garlic, cooking wine, teriyaki sauce, garlic salt, and black pepper in the hot oil and butter until mushrooms are lightly browned, about 5 minutes. Reduce heat to low and simmer until mushrooms are tender, 5 to 8 more minutes.[91,92]

91 Veronika Weaver1, Keith Martin2, and Margherita T Cantorna1, "The Effects of Whole Mushrooms during Inflammation," BMC Immunology (BioMed Central, February 20, 2009), http://bmcimmunol.biomedcentral.com/articles/10.1186/1471-2172-10-12.

92 K R Martin and S K Brophy, "Commonly Consumed and Specialty Dietary Mushrooms Reduce Cellular Proliferation in MCF-7 Human Breast Cancer Cells.," Experimental biology and medicine (Maywood, N.J.). (U.S. National Library of Medicine, November 2010), https://www.ncbi.nlm.nih.gov/pubmed?term=crimini mushroom breast cancer.

68. NUTRITIONAL YEAST

The Why:

Nutritional yeast has several benefits. One of the biggest benefits of nutritional yeast is that it is often high in B12, an important vitamin that much of the population is deficient in. The B12 in yeast is either included as an additive at the end of its manufacture, or else the yeast is grown in a B12-enriched medium. The latter method is best because it incorporates the vitamin into the living food. Some nutritional yeasts do not contain vitamin B12; to be sure, check the list of nutrients on the container.

Aside from B12, nutritional yeast is also a "complete protein," it contains other B vitamins, is low in fat and sodium, is free of sugar and gluten, and contains iron.

The Science:

In an article by Dr. Alan Christianson, N.D., published in Nutrition Science News, he reports that nutritional yeast provides a significant dose of important minerals, such as iron. This is particularly important to help athletes who train more than four hours per week prevent iron deficiency. Nutritional yeast also contains selenium, which helps repair cell damage, and benefit-rich zinc, which aids in tissue repair, wound healing, and maintains our sense of taste and smell.

Fortified nutritional yeast has significantly less iron than the unfortified type, however. Elizabeth Brown, a registered dietitian and certified holistic chef specializing in weight management, sports nutrition, disease prevention and optimizing health through whole foods, reports that "beta-1,3 glucan, is a type of fiber that may aid the immune system and help to lower cholesterol. Additionally, nutritional yeast is a good source of selenium and potassium."

Thus, nutritional yeast may help lower cholesterol naturally and also naturally treat cancer due to its selenium content.

The How:

Nutritional yeast can usually be found in the bulk or supplement sections of health food stores, though you may lose some of the nutritional value of the riboflavin since it is light sensitive.

Though it is most popular among vegans and vegetarians, nutritional yeast is delicious, adding amazing flavor and nutrition without the high fat and calories associated with cheese. For those who are lactose intolerant, nutritional yeast is a perfect choice because it can be sprinkled on pasta, salads, baked or mashed potatoes, soups, and even popcorn![93]

[93] Rachael Link, "The Antiviral, Antibacterial Immune-Booster," Dr. Axe, April 24, 2019, https://draxe.com/nutritional-yeast/.

69. OLIVE OIL

The Why:

Olive oil is nature's vitamin E, aka antioxidant.. When you use olive oil as a dressing it retains its health benefits. Cooking with it at a high heat turns the oil rancid and into a free radical causing cell damage. Keep the high heat cooking to coconut oil and enjoy olive oil as a dressing.

The Science:

Investigators at the University of Monastir, Tunisia, and King Saud University, Saudi Arabia, carried out a study demonstrating that extra virgin olive oil may protect the liver from oxidative stress. Oxidative stress refers to the cell damage associated with the chemical reaction between free radicals and other molecules in the body. Put simply, oxidative stress means cell damage.

In this study, which was published in BioMed Central, Mohamed Hammami and colleagues reported that laboratory rats exposed to a moderately toxic herbicide that were fed on a diet containing olive oil were partially protected from liver damage.

Hammami said "Olive oil is an integral ingredient in the Mediterranean diet. There is growing evidence that it may have great health benefits including the reduction in coronary heart disease risk, the prevention of some cancers and the modification of immune and inflammatory responses. Here, we've shown that extra virgin olive oil and its extracts protect against oxidative damage of hepatic tissue."[94]

[94] "Olive Oil Protects Liver," Medical News Today (MediLexicon International, October 29, 2010), http://www.medicalnewstoday.com/releases/206092.php.

The How:

Using Olive Oil

1. Drizzle it over salad or mix it into a homemade salad dressing.
2. Use in marinades or sauces for meat, fish, poultry, and vegetables.
3. Add at the end of cooking for a burst of flavor.
4. Drizzle over cooked vegetables.[95]

[95] Gayle A. Alleman, "Ultimate Guide to Olive Oil," HowStuffWorks (HowStuffWorks, December 27, 2006), http://recipes.howstuffworks.com/how-olive-oil-works4.htm.

70. ONIONS

The Why:

Onions do more than add flavor your favorite dish. They are low in calories, have virtually no fat and are loaded with healthful components that fight inflammation in arthritis and related conditions.

The Science:

Onions boost circulation and immunity. They contain sulfides, which lower blood pressure & lipids (fats). Research at Tufts has shown that onions raise HDL (good cholesterol) by as much as 30%.

Onions are also one of the richest sources of flavonoids, antioxidants that mop up free radicals in your body's cells before they have a chance to cause harm. One flavonoid found in onions, called quercetin, has been shown to inhibit inflammation-causing leukotrienes, prostaglandins and histamines in osteoarthritis (OA) and rheumatoid arthritis (RA), reduce heart disease risk by lowering low-density lipoprotein (LDL) or "bad" cholesterol and help prevent the progression of cancer.

The How:

Dice the perfect onion:

1. Cut the onion in half, slicing downwards through the root, then peel.
2. Cut 5-6 vertical slices into each half, leaving the root intact.
3. Lay the onion half flat, slicing horizontally and keeping the root intact.
4. Slice downwards across these cuts to dice.[96]

[96] Waitrose Limited, "How to Dice an Onion," How to dice an onion - Step by step - Recipes - Waitrose.com, accessed October 1, 2019, http://www.waitrose.com/home/recipes/step_by_step/how_to_dice_an_onion.html.

71. FREE-RANGE CHICKEN

The Why:

One of the healthiest benefits of free-range chicken is its high protein content. Just one free-range chicken breast can supply around 52% of most people's daily protein needs. Protein is crucial to the health of our bodies. It's so crucial in fact it's even referred to as "the building block of life." When you don't get an adequate amount of protein in your diet, your cells have a more difficult time growing and repairing themselves. For growing kids and pregnant women with growing babies, protein is especially vital.

The Science:

A scientific study published in 2017 looked at the effects of feeding commercial chicken feed, conventional chicken meat or organic chicken meat to groups of female animal subjects. To evaluate the effects, researchers took measurements of the subjects' percent growth rate and cholesterol levels as well as their levels of progesterone, testosterone and estrogen levels.

They discovered that consuming both commercial chicken feed and commercial chicken meat resulted in increases in growth, increases in cholesterol levels and an imbalance in hormone levels. Overall, the study concludes that "commercial chicken feed and commercial chicken meat may be the potential cause of development of polycystic ovary syndrome in females due to steroid hormonal imbalance."

The How:

How to Find Free-Range Chicken:

If you have a local farm or farmers market, then getting free-range chicken from a supplier close to your home is always a great way to go. With a locally sourced free-range chicken, you are likely to get much fresher meat. Plus, you may even be able to visit the farm and see exactly how the chickens live on a daily basis.

Health stores that carry chicken products typically only carry chicken that is organic or organic and free-range. Nowadays, it's also easy to find free-range chicken in your grocery store. With all the problems with conventional chicken, it has definitely become easier to find free-range and organic chicken in many locations.[97,98]

[97] "Simple Baked Chicken Breasts," Allrecipes, accessed October 1, 2019, http://allrecipes.com/recipe/240208/simple-baked-chicken-breasts/.

[98] Saara Ahmad et al., "Daily Consumption of Commercial Chicken Feed and Meat Lead to Alterations in Serum Cholesterol and Steroidal Sex Hormones in Female Rats," Pakistan journal of pharmaceutical sciences (U.S. National Library of Medicine, January 2017), https://www.ncbi.nlm.nih.gov/pubmed/28625952.

72. OYSTERS

The Why:

It's beneficial to include something raw in your diet and oysters are a great way to go.

The impressive health benefits of oysters come from their vast stockpiles of minerals, vitamins, and organic compounds. In fact, certain mineral varieties are in their highest content in oysters, meaning that they are the premiere food item in the entire world for supplementation, particularly of zinc. We don't get enough zinc in our diet through veggies alone and oysters are a great way to increase this mineral in our bodies. Of the trace minerals zinc is only second to iron.

The Science:

Oysters really are an aphrodisiac...sort of. Very few scientific studies have shown that oysters can actually raise your sexual desire, but they still may help spur it on. Oysters contain more zinc per serving than any other food; zinc is a key mineral for sexual health in men, and severe cases of zinc deficiency can lead to impotence. However, it's more likely that oysters could raise your libido by the power of suggestion, much like peaches, alcohol, chocolate, or any other food with a desire-boosting reputation.[99]

[99] Adam Lusher, "Raw Oysters Really Are Aphrodisiacs Say Scientists (and Now Is the Time to Eat Them)," The Telegraph (Telegraph Media Group, March 20, 2005), http://www.telegraph.co.uk/news/uknews/1486054/Raw-oysters-really-are-aphrodisiacs-say-scientists-and-now-is-the-time-to-eat-them.html.

The How:

Start by sorting through your oysters and selecting the ones which are tightly closed. Discard any oysters which have opened, as these are dead and are no longer suitable for eating.

Give the oysters a quick wash before serving them.

Hold the oyster down with a cloth against a flat surface.

Using an oyster knife with a hand guard, insert the tip of the knife into the small hole at the hinge of the oyster shell. Wiggle the knife and push it all the way inside the shell to break the hinge.

Angle the knife upwards as you push it in, so that you cut the abductor muscle which holds the oyster onto the top shell. Remove the top shell, keeping the bottom shell flat to conserve the oyster juices. Then cut the abductor muscle holding the oyster onto the bottom shell so that it is lying loose on the shell, ready for serving.

Serve the oysters immediately on a bed of crushed ice.

Pick the oyster shell up, keeping it flat so as not to spill the juices. Hold it so that the smooth edge of the shell is facing towards you.

Tip the shell up and let the oyster and its juices slide into your mouth.[100,101]

[100] Person and wikiHow, "How to Eat Oysters," wikiHow (wikiHow, September 6, 2019), http://www.wikihow.com/Eat-Oysters.

[101] John Staughton and John Staughton, "8 Wonderful Benefits of Oysters," Organic Facts, July 12, 2019, https://www.organicfacts.net/health-benefits/animal-product/oysters.html.

73. PINK HIMALAYAN SALT

The Why:

Himalayan salt contains 84 trace minerals that your body needs, as well as electrolytes your cells need for energy production. Plus, it makes your food taste yummy.

Himalayan Crystal Salt contains the same 84 natural minerals and elements found in the human body. This form of salt has also matured over the past 250 million years under intense tectonic pressure, creating an environment of zero exposure to toxins and impurities.

Himalayan salt's unique cellular structure allows it to store vibrational energy. Its minerals exist in a colloidal form, meaning that they are tiny enough for our cells to easily absorb.

The Science:

Pink Himalayan salt is a much more balanced and healthy choice in comparison to common table salt. True, high-quality pink Himalayan salt is one of the purest salts you can find. It's even typically mined by hand. This is very different from table salt that involves a great deal of unnatural interference. Table salt is very heavily processed, eliminating its minerals. Commercial table salt is typically 97.5%to 99.9% sodium chloride. Meanwhile, a high-quality unrefined salt like Himalayan sea salt is only about 87% sodium chloride.

With most table salts, you're only left with one mineral, sodium. Some brands add iodine and other really health-hazardous anti-clumping agents, like yellow prussiate of soda. Many commercial table salts also undergo a bleaching process and contain aluminum derivatives and other terrible ingredients known to be highly toxic to human health.

The How:

You should always store salt in an airtight, covered container in a cool, dry place to keep it at its best. The only true source of real Himalayan salt is Pakistan, so make sure to check your labels. I would stay away from any "Himalayan salt" that's sold at a lower price point. This may be a sign that the salt was collected from higher elevations rather from the deeper, more pure salt mines. The salts from these higher levels are more likely to contain impurities, which makes them less health-promoting.

Since pink Himalayan salt contains so many minerals, it's more beneficial to the body, but as a salt, it's still naturally high in sodium. So as with any salt, you don't want to overdo it. Getting too much sodium in the diet (especially with not enough potassium to balance things out) can lead to high blood pressure for some people. It can also lead to a concerning buildup of fluid in people with congestive heart failure, cirrhosis of the liver or kidney disease.

74. PUMPKINS

The Why:

Got digestive issues? Try eating pumpkin. The fiber in pumpkin is helpful for all digestive problems, including IBS and diarrhea which respond well to cooked pumpkin.

Pumpkins are a type of squash that grow all over the United States and is easily found at local farmers markets, roadside vegetable stands and organic produce delivery services. Pumpkins are rich in nutritional benefits and can be used in a wide variety of dishes. Add it to stews, salads and soups to avail yourself of this nutritious vegetable.

The Science:

As part of the squash family, pumpkins are especially rich in the pigments lutein and zeaxanthin. A 2008 study followed more than 35,000 women for an average of 10 years. Those with the highest amounts of these two pigments in their diet (6,716 mcg per day) had an 18% lower risk of cataracts compared to those with the lowest (1,177 mcg per day). One cup (250 mL) of cooked pumpkin has 2,484 mcg.

The How:

- Preheat oven to 400 degrees F (200 degrees C).
- Peel and cube pumpkin.
- Toss with olive oil and garlic in a large bowl.
- Season with salt and black pepper.
- Arrange coated pumpkin on a baking sheet.
- Roast in the preheated oven until squash is tender and lightly browned, 25 to 30 minutes.[102]

[102] "Simple Roasted Butternut Squash Recipe," Allrecipes, December 22, 2012, http://allrecipes.com/recipe/229733/simple-roasted-butternut-squash/.

75. PUMPKIN SEEDS

The Why:

Pumpkin seeds are nature's mineral healer. One the richest sources of zinc make it very beneficial for men with an enlarged prostate. They have also been shown to reduce inflammation and help with arthritis-type conditions.

The Science:

Pumpkin seeds have long been valued as a source of the mineral zinc, and the World Health Organization recommends their consumption as a good way of obtaining this nutrient. If you want to maximize the amount of zinc that you get from your pumpkin seeds, we recommend that you purchase them in unshelled form. Although recent studies have shown there to be little zinc in the shell itself, zinc is especially concentrated in the endosperm envelope. Because it can be tricky to separate the endosperm envelope from the shell, eating the entire pumpkin seed—shell and all—will ensure that all of the zinc-containing portions of the seed are consumed. Whole roasted, unshelled pumpkin seeds contain about 10 milligrams of zinc per 3.5 ounces, and shelled roasted pumpkin seeds (which are often referred to pumpkin seed kernels) contain about 7 to 8 milligrams. So even though the difference is not huge, and the seed kernels remain a good source of zinc, you'll be able to increase your zinc intake if you consume the unshelled version.

The How:

When roasting pumpkin seeds at home, it is recommended you roast them for no more than 15 to 20 minutes. This recommendation is supported by a new study that pinpointed 20 minutes as a threshold time for changes in pumpkin seed fats. In this recent study, pumpkin seeds were roasted in a microwave oven for varying lengths of time, and limited changes in the pumpkin seeds fat were determined to occur under 20 minutes. However, when the seeds were roasted for longer than 20 minutes, a number of unwanted changes in fat structure were determined to occur more frequently.

76. RAW MILK

The Why:

Raw milk has all the enzymes and nutrients needed to be considered a complete food. The health benefits have been associated with healthier skin, hair and nails, better absorption of nutrients, a stronger immune system, reduced allergies, and increased bone density.

The Science:

Studies show that children fed raw milk have more resistance to TB than children fed pasteurized milk; that raw milk is very effective in preventing scurvy and protecting against the flu, diphtheria and pneumonia; that raw milk prevents tooth decay, even in children who eat a lot of sugar; that raw milk is better than pasteurized milk in promoting growth and calcium absorption; that a substance present in raw cream (but not in pasteurized cream) prevents joint stiffness and the pain of arthritis; and that children who drink raw milk have fewer skin allergies and far less asthma than children who drink pasteurized milk.

The How:

Drinking raw milk is like being a journalist, make sure you know & trust your sources.

Raw dairy isn't always easy to find, since laws differ from state to state regarding consumers' rights to buy raw milk.

For a summary of state laws on selling real, raw milk, visit the website: https://www.realmilk.com/, specifically, the Raw Milk Nation map on the State Updates page. In summary, raw milk can be sold in stores in ten states and purchased at the farm in about 28 states. Raw milk is available as pet food in four states, and through cow- and herd-share agreements in several other states.[103,104,105,106,107,108]

[103] Webmaster Realmilk.com, "Abstracts on the Effect of Pasteurization on the Nutritional Value...," A Campaign for Real Milk, February 4, 2014, https://www.realmilk.com/health/abstracts-on-the-effect-of-pasteurization/.

[104] Thompson S. Westcott and Frederick O. Waage, "Observations on the Presence of Bacillus Abortus Bovinus in Certified Milk (Preliminary Notes)," The American Journal of the Medical Sciences 154, no. 5 (1917): p. 767, https://doi.org/10.1097/00000441-191711000-00023.

[105] "List of Bulletins of the Ohio Agricultural Experiment Station, Wooster, Ohio [1944]," KB Home (Ohio Agricultural Experiment Station, January 1, 1970), https://kb.osu.edu/handle/1811/71988.

[106] "Annual Review of Biochemistry," annualreviews.org, accessed October 2, 2019, https://www.annualreviews.org/toc/biochem/18/1.

[107] Josef Riedler et al., "Exposure to Farming in Early Life and Development of Asthma and Allergy: a Cross-Sectional Survey," The Lancet 358, no. 9288 (2001): pp. 1129-1133, https://doi.org/10.1016/s0140-6736(01)06252-3.

[108] Georg Loss and Silvia Apprich, "The Protective Effect of Farm Milk Consumption on Childhood Asthma and Atopy: The GABRIELA Study," The Journal of Allergy and Clinical Immunology, October 2011, http://www.jacionline.org/article/S0091-6749(11)01234-6/abstract.

77. ROSEMARY

The Why:

Use more herbs in your cooking like rosemary. The most interesting and unique health benefits of rosemary include its ability to boost memory, improve mood, reduce inflammation, relieve pain, protect the immune system, stimulate circulation, detoxify the body, protect the body from bacterial infections, prevent premature aging, and heal skin conditions.

The Science:

Neurological protection scientists have found that rosemary is also good for your brain. Rosemary contains an ingredient, carnosic acid, that is able to fight off free radical damage in the brain. According to a study published in Cell Journal, carnosic acid "may be useful in protecting against beta amyloid-induced neurodegeneration in the hippocampus."

The How:

Whenever possible, choose fresh rosemary over the dried form of the herb since it is far superior in flavor. Sprigs of fresh rosemary look vibrantly fresh, are deep sage green in color, and free from yellow or dark spots.

Even though dried herbs and spices are widely available in supermarkets, explore the local spice stores in your area. Oftentimes, these stores feature an expansive selection of dried herbs and spices that are of superior quality and freshness to those offered in regular markets. Just like with other dried herbs, when purchasing dried rosemary, try to select organically grown herbs since this will give you more assurance that the herbs contain no pesticide residues and have not been irradiated (among other potential adverse effects, irradiating rosemary may lead to a significant decrease in its carotenoid content.)

Fresh rosemary should be stored in the refrigerator either in its original packaging or wrapped in a slightly damp paper towel. You can also place the rosemary sprigs in ice cube trays covered with either water or stock that can then be added when preparing soups or stews. Dried rosemary should be kept in a tightly sealed container in a cool, dark and dry place where it will keep fresh for about six months.[109,110]

[109] Joseph Nordqvist, "Rosemary: Health Benefits, Precautions, and Drug Interactions," Medical News Today (MediLexicon International, December 13, 2017), http://www.medicalnewstoday.com/articles/266370.php.

[110] "Rosemary," The World's Healthiest Foods, accessed October 1, 2019, http://www.whfoods.com/genpage.php?tname=foodspice&dbid=75.

78. SAGE

The Why:

Sage gets its name from the Latin word salvere, which means "to save." During the middle ages, sage had a strong reputation for its healing properties, and was even used to help prevent the plague. Adding fresh herbs to your cooking will deepen the flavor profile.

The Science:

Sage can improve brain function and memory. Current research indicates that sage may be able to improve brain function and memory, especially in people with Alzheimer's disease. Sage inhibits the breakdown of acetylcholine, a chemical messenger in the brain. Drops in levels of this chemical are seen in those suffering from Alzheimer's disease.

The How:

Whenever possible, choose fresh sage over the dried form of the herb since it is superior in flavor. The leaves of fresh sage look fresh and are a vibrant greenish-gray in color. They should be free from darks spots or yellowing.

To store fresh sage leaves, carefully wrap them in a damp paper towel and place inside a loosely closed plastic bag. Store in the refrigerator where it should keep fresh for several days. Dried sage should be kept in a tightly sealed glass container in a cool, dark and dry place where it will keep fresh for about six months.[111]

[111] Nicolette S L Perry et al., "Salvia for Dementia Therapy: Review of Pharmacological Activity and Pilot Tolerability Clinical Trial," Pharmacology, biochemistry, and behavior (U.S. National Library of Medicine, June 2003), https://www.ncbi.nlm.nih.gov/pubmed/12895683.

79. MAKE YOUR OWN SALAD DRESSING

The Why:

The vast majority of commercial salad dressings are far from healthy. They are full of high fructose corn syrup and highly processed omega-6 GMO oils that contain toxic herbicides like glyphosate. You should also avoid low-fat dressings. When fat is removed from a food product, it's usually replaced by sugar/fructose in order to make that food taste good, and this is a recipe for poor health. Excess fructose in your diet drives insulin and leptin resistance, which are at the heart of not only diabetes but most other chronic diseases as well.

The Science:

Scientists recently discovered that eating a high-fructose diet for just six weeks may make you less smart. While you expect high-fructose corn syrup in foods like candy, you may be surprised to find it in many popular salad dressings and high-end brands.

Salad dressings also have hidden deadly fats. Trans fats are dangerous industrialized fats that your taste buds love but your body hates, thanks to the ingredients tendency to promote heart disease. Used to help extend a product's shelf life, trans fats are required to be listed on labels, but there's a loophole - foods that contain less than .5 grams of trans fat per serving are not required to list trans fats on the label, and food manufacturers are capitalizing on it.

You can recognize the presence of trans fats that are not listed on labels by looking for ingredients containing "partially hydrogenated," "shortening," or "interesterified." To reduce the time it takes to read the fine print, just grab an organic dressing, where trans fats and many other toxic ingredients, are banned, or better yet, make your own!

The How:

Make Your Own Basic Salad Dressing

INGREDIENTS

- 8 tablespoons olive oil
- 2 tablespoons Balsamic vinegar (raw is optimal)
- 1 tablespoon Red Wine Vinegar (raw is optimal)
- Sea salt and pepper to taste

INSTRUCTIONS

Whisk ingredients together in a bowl well.

We store ours in a glass bottle (usually a recycled one from olive oil or vinegar) in the cupboard. Some people store theirs in the refrigerator, but if you do, you will have to take it out about 20 to 30 minutes before using it to allow the olive oil to soften – as olive oil will harden when cooled. A trick we use is to add a small amount of sustainable-produced, cold-pressed grapeseed oil to keep the dressing from hardening.

80. SARDINES

The Why:

Sardines are one of the highest sources of essential omega-3 fatty acids on the planet, and they include many other important trace minerals and vitamins. Due to their size they have the least amount of mercury compared to bigger fish and are an inexpensive healthy snack.

The Science:

Sardines are one of the best natural sources in the world of essential omega-3 fatty acids, with one 3.2 oz can providing roughly 50% of your daily needs. Sardines provide both EPA and DHA, which are two fatty acids that studies show the body uses to reduce inflammation, resulting in improved heart health, the ability to maintain proper brain function and ward off gum disease, and much more.

The How:

Sardines with Sun-Dried Tomato and Capers

- Place the sardines on a small plate.
- Squeeze the lemon half over the sardines.
- Season with salt, black pepper, cayenne pepper, oregano, thyme, and crushed red pepper flakes.
- Scatter the garlic, sun-dried tomatoes, and capers over the mixture.[112,113]

[112] Jaime, "Sardines with Sun-Dried Tomato and Capers Recipe," Allrecipes, July 15, 2011, http://allrecipes.com/recipe/218369/sardines-with-sun-dried-tomato-and-capers/?internalSource=hn_carousel 01_Sardines with Tomatoes and Capers&referringId=13337&referringContentType=recipe hub&referringPosition=carousel 01.

[113] Joseph Charles Maroon and Jeffrey W Bost, "Omega-3 Fatty Acids (Fish Oil) as an Anti-Inflammatory: an Alternative to Nonsteroidal Anti-Inflammatory Drugs for Discogenic Pain," Surgical neurology (U.S. National Library of Medicine, April 2006), https://www.ncbi.nlm.nih.gov/pubmed/16531187.

81. SAUERKRAUT

The Why:

A forkful of sauerkraut helps the probiotics go down. Fermented cabbage has a powerful phytochemical called DIM that is both fights cancer and strengthens the gut. The goal with probiotics is to get them alive in food so you have more of the good guys fighting off the bad guys.

The Science:

In 2005, a team of researchers from Poland and the United states observed a substantially higher rate of breast cancer among Polish women who immigrated to the United States. They compared Polish women who were living in and near Chicago and Detroit with women who were still living in Poland. They observed that the rate of breast cancer was three times higher for the Polish immigrants. They evaluated various factors and concluded that the consumption of lacto-fermented sauerkraut was a possible factor in the different cancer rates. Women in Poland ate an average of 30 pounds of raw sauerkraut each year, while the Polish women in the U.S. ate approximately 10 pounds per year.[114,115]

[114] "Sauerkraut: Anti-Cancer Fermented Food That Restores Gut Flora," Health Impact News, January 27, 2017, https://healthimpactnews.com/2014/sauerkraut-anti-cancer-fermented-food-that-restores-gut-flora/.

[115] Dominique Patton, "Sauerkraut Consumption May Fight off Breast Cancer," nutraingredients.com (William Reed Business Media Ltd., November 4, 2005), https://www.nutraingredients.com/Research/Sauerkraut-consumption-may-fight-off-breast-cancer.

The How:

Homemade Sauerkraut

HOMEMADE SAUERKRAUT RECIPE

INGREDIENTS:

1 Medium Head of Cabbage
1-3 Tbsp. sea salt

INSTRUCTIONS:

- Chop or shred cabbage. Sprinkle with salt.
- Knead the cabbage with clean hands, or pound with a potato masher or Cabbage Crusher about 10 minutes, until there is enough liquid to cover.
- Stuff the cabbage into a quart jar, pressing the cabbage underneath the liquid. If necessary, add a bit of water to completely cover cabbage.
- Cover the jar with a tight lid, airlock lid, or coffee filter secured with a rubber band.
- Culture at room temperature (60-70°F is preferred) for at least 2 weeks until desired flavor and texture are achieved. If using a tight lid, burp daily to release excess pressure.
- Once the sauerkraut is finished, put a tight lid on the jar and move to cold storage. The sauerkraut's flavor will continue to develop as it ages.[116]

[116] "Cultures For Health," Cultures for Health, accessed October 1, 2019, http://www.culturesforhealth.com/learn/recipe/natural-fermentation/sauerkraut/.

82. SEA VEGETABLES

The Why:

Seaweed and sea vegetables contain all 56 elements essential for human health, including calcium, magnesium, potassium, iodine, iron, and zinc, together with important trace elements such as selenium that are often lacking in land vegetables due to soil demineralisation.

The Science:

Dr. Jane Teas of Harvard University published a paper proposing that kelp (kombu and wakame) consumption may be a factor in the lower rates of breast cancer seen in Japan compared to the United States. She is now researching the effects of sea vegetables as a natural alternative to HRT (hormone replacement therapy). Sea vegetables are very high in lignans, plant substances that become phytoestrogens in the body, meaning that they help to block the chemical oestrogens that can predispose people to cancers such as breast cancer.

The How:

Identifying the most common sea vegetables:

- Arame - mild and sweet, lacy and wiry sea vegetable.
- Dulse - chewy and soft seaweed.
- Hijiki - strong-flavored sea vegetable that looks like wiry, black pasta.
- Kelp - varies from light brown to dark green in color.
- Kombu - sold as a soup flavoring and is very dark.
- Nori - purple-black variety of seaweed and turns green when toasted. Also the one we are most familiar with for its use in sushi rolls.
- Wakame - sold in strips or sheets like Kombu and is often used to flavor soups.[117]

[117] Annie Price, "Taking 1 Gram of This Daily by Mouth for a Year Reduces Pre-Cancerous Mouth Sores," Dr. Axe, November 23, 2016, https://draxe.com/simplifying-sea-vegetables/.

83. SOAKED NUTS

The Why:

Soaking nuts helps to break down enzymes, lactobacilli, and other helpful organisms and neutralize a large portion of phytic acid in nuts. Soaking in warm water also neutralizes enzyme inhibitors, present in all seeds, and encourages the production of numerous beneficial enzymes. The action of these enzymes also increases the amount of many vitamins, especially B vitamins. During the process of soaking and fermenting, gluten and other difficult-to-digest proteins are partially broken down into simpler components that are more readily available for absorption.

The Science:

Soaked almonds are known to help greatly improve a person's digestive system. In a study published in the Journal of Food Science, it was found that eating raw, soaked almonds helped empty the stomach faster and made digesting proteins easier. Apart from that, the fact that the almonds are soaked deactivates the enzyme inhibiting compound (found on the skin of the almond) and initiates the release of an essential lipase, that helps in the proper breakdown of fat; therefore improving the digestion and absorption of nutrients.

The How:

Traditional soaked nuts and seeds, are made by following these basic steps:

1. Measure out 4 cups of raw, unsalted, organic nuts/seeds into a medium sized bowl.
2. Cover with filtered water so that nuts are submerged.
3. Add 1-2 tablespoons unrefined salt.
4. Allow to stand covered on the counter for about 7 hours, or overnight.
5. Rinse nuts to remove salt residue and spread out in single layer on a rack to dehydrate.
6. Dry at a low temperature (generally no higher than 150°F, although there are exceptions) in dehydrator or oven for 12-24 hours or until nuts are slightly crispy.[118,119,120]

[118] Kayla Grossmann, "That's Nuts! A Complete Guide to Soaking Nuts and Seeds," That's Nuts! A Complete Guide to Soaking Nuts and Seeds, accessed October 1, 2019, http://blog.radiantlifecatalog.com/bid/69542/That-s-Nuts-A-Complete-Guide-to-Soaking-Nuts-and-Seeds.

[119] Gail M. Bornhorst et al., "Gastric Digestion of Raw and Roasted AlmondsIn Vivo," Journal of Food Science 78, no. 11 (August 2013), https://doi.org/10.1111/1750-3841.12274.

[120] Chung-Yen Chen, Karen Lapsley, and Jeffrey Blumberg, "A Nutrition and Health Perspective on Almonds," Journal of the Science of Food and Agriculture 86, no. 14 (2006): pp. 2245-2250, https://doi.org/10.1002/jsfa.2659.

84. SPROUTED BREAD

The Why:

Sprouted bread is a great solution for people that want to include bread in their healthy lifestyle. Sprouted bread comes from grains that have been germinated and allowed to sprout green buds. The sprouted grain process involves soaking the grains in water until they begin to grow a sprout. The growing environment is highly controlled, including the water temp, air temp, and the time grains are allowed to sprout. Once the grains sprout, they are drained and mixed together to be ground up and used. Before the sprouted grain is used, it is a living food. Enzymes are released during the sprouting process, which break down proteins and carbohydrates. This process helps make sprouted grain food low glycemic and easier to digest.

To get the full health benefits, add grassfed butter. The vitamin A in the butter helps you absorb and activate the B vitamins.

The Science:

Sprouted Bread studies show that sprouting grains increases their content of the amino acid lysine. Lysine is the limiting amino acid in many plants, so sprouting increases the efficiency that the proteins in the grain can be used for structural and functional purposes in the human body.[121]

---

[121] "Figure 2f from: Irimia R, Gottschling M (2016) Taxonomic Revision of Rochefortia Sw. (Ehretiaceae, Boraginales). Biodiversity Data Journal 4: e7720. Https://Doi.org/10.3897/BDJ.4.e7720," Changes in the Carbohydrates and Nitrogenous Components during Germination of Proso Millet, Panicum Miliaceum. 45 (n.d.), https://doi.org/10.3897/bdj.4.e7720.figure2f.

The How:

When buying sprouted bread look for it in the refrigerated section at your health food store. My favorite sprouted grain bread is the classic – Ezekiel 4:9 Sprouted Grain Bread by Food for Life – it's made from six different organic sprouted grains and absolutely no flour! This combo of sprouted grains contains all nine essential amino acids, which makes up a complete protein.

Other good sprouted breads are Manna's Sunseed bread and Dave's Killer Bread Sprouted Wheat, which are both a healthy combo of organic sprouted wheat and seeds.[122]

122 Food Babe, "Before You Ever Buy Bread Again...Read This! (And Find The Healthiest Bread On The Market)," Food Babe, July 24, 2017, http://foodbabe.com/2014/02/24/healthiest-bread-on-the-market/.

85. SPROUTS

The Why:

Sprouts are known as a nutritional powerhouse. They have highly concentrated nutritional benefits compared to mature vegetables. Sprouts are low in calories and rich in fiber, enzymes, protein, and other micronutrients. The health benefits of sprouts make up quite an impressive list, and they include the ability to improve the digestive process, boost the metabolism, increase enzymatic activity throughout the body, prevent anemia, aid in weight loss, lower cholesterol, reduce blood pressure, prevent neural tube defects in infants, boost skin health, improve vision, support the immune system, and increase usable energy reserves.

The Science:

Sprouts are a great source of omega-3 fatty acids, and although these are technically a form of cholesterol, they are considered "good" cholesterol (HDL cholesterol) and can actually reduce the amount of harmful cholesterol in your blood vessels and arteries. A study by The Center for Genetics in Washington D.C., confirmed that sprouts are high in antioxidants and omega-3. The omega-3 fatty acids are also anti-inflammatory in nature, so they reduce the stress on your cardiovascular system as well. The potassium content of sprouts also helps to reduce blood pressure, since potassium is a vasodilator, and can release the tension in arteries and blood vessels. This increases circulation and oxygenation while reducing clotting and lowering the risk of atherosclerosis, heart attacks, and strokes.

The How:

- Wash hands well and make sure that all equipment is clean and sterile.
- Pour one type of seed into quart size jar. Use about 1 teaspoon of small seeds like alfalfa or broccoli or 1/4 cup of beans and lentils.
- Cover with 1 cup of filtered water and put lid or cheesecloth over the jar.
- Allow to soak for up to 12 hours. It is often easiest to soak overnight.
- In the morning, strain off the water. This is easily done with a sprouting lid. If you are using a cheesecloth, strain through a fine strainer and return to jar.
- Rinse well with filtered water and drain again.
- Place upside down at a slight angle so that excess water can drain off and air can get in. I find a dish rack or medium size bowl is perfect for this.
- Re-rinse the sprouts several times a day with filtered water, returning to the tilted position each time.
- You should see sprouting in a day or two, with most sprouts ready to harvest in 3-7 days.
- When done sprouting, rinse thoroughly in cool, filtered water and store in a covered container in the fridge for up to a week.

Sprouts can be easily added to your table, by adding them to salads, soups, sandwiches, stir-fries, sautéed vegetables, pastas and smoothies.[123],[124]

123 Katie Wells and Katie Wells, "How to Grow Sprouts at Home: Wellness Mama," Wellness Mama®, July 30, 2019, https://wellnessmama.com/36686/how-to-grow-sprouts/.

124 ARTEMIS SIMOPOULOS, "Omega-3 Fatty Acids and Antioxidants in Edible Wild Plants," November 3, 2002, https://scielo.conicyt.cl/pdf/bres/v37n2/art13.pdf.

86. SQUASH

The Why:

Squash is called a 'warming food' in Chinese medicine. These vegetables bring heat into the body which is why we eat them particularly in colder months. People with low blood pressure will find it helps them stay warm by improving blood circulation.

The Science:

Squash is an important source for immune system health. It contains many nutrients, including vitamin C, magnesium, and other antioxidant compounds. These vitamins and minerals are important antioxidant components in the body, and help to neutralize free radicals throughout the body. Free radicals are the natural, dangerous byproducts of cellular metabolism, and they have been connected with a wide swath of illnesses, including cancer, heart disease, and premature aging. Furthermore, squash contains very high levels of vitamin A, including carotenoid phytonutrients like lutein and zeaxanthin. All of this together helps the body to boost its immune response and defend against the foreign substances, as well as the free radicals produced by our own body, that may do us harm over the long term.[125]

[125] John Staughton, "7 Amazing Benefits of Squash," Organic Facts, July 3, 2019, https://www.organicfacts.net/health-benefits/fruit/squash.html.

The How:

Easy Butternut Squash Recipe:

- Preheat oven to 400 degrees F (200 degrees C).
- Peel butternut squash and cut into small cubes.
- Toss butternut squash with olive oil and garlic in a large bowl.
- Season with salt and black pepper.
- Arrange coated squash on a baking sheet.
- Roast in the preheated oven until squash is tender and lightly browned, 25 to 30 minutes.

87. TOMATOES

The Why:

The health benefits of tomatoes include eye care, good stomach health, and reduced blood pressure. They provide relief from diabetes, skin problems, and urinary tract infections too. Furthermore, they improve digestion, stimulate blood circulation, reduce cholesterol levels, improve fluid balance, protect the kidneys, detoxify the body, prevent premature aging, and reduce inflammation. Tomatoes consist of a large number of antioxidants which may help fight different types of cancer. They are also a rich source of vitamins and minerals which provide protection against cardiovascular diseases.

The Science:

Tomatoes contain a large amount of lycopene which is a carotenoid and an antioxidant that is highly effective in scavenging cancer-causing free radicals. This benefit can even be obtained from heat-processed tomato products like homemade ketchup. The lycopene in tomatoes defends against cancer and has been shown to be effective in fighting prostate cancer, according to a study led by Dr. Edward Giovannucci of the Harvard School of Public Health. Another study suggests that lycopene may help prevent the growth of prostate and breast cancer cells. The results of an animal study suggest that lycopene has the potential to prevent renal cell cancer.

Further scientific studies and evidence is required to support the anticancer potential of lycopene.

The How:

You can incorporate tomatoes into your diet in a number of forms—fresh, dried, or as sauce, salsa, or paste. Add fresh tomatoes to omelets and salads, or serve them sliced, drizzled with balsamic and garnished with fresh basil, sea salt, and cracked black pepper. Dress fresh greens or steamed veggies with sundried tomato pesto, or drizzle it over broiled fish. Toss spaghetti squash or beans with tomato sauce, or use it as a topping for sautéed green beans or potatoes. Add salsa to scrambled eggs or taco salad, or spoon onto cooked fish, black beans, or brown rice. Use tomato paste in veggie chili, or mix it into hummus, along with roasted garlic and harissa.[126,127]

[126] Christine Gallary, "3 Essential Tips for Cutting Tomatoes," Kitchn (Apartment Therapy, LLC., May 2, 2019), http://www.thekitchn.com/3-essential-tips-for-cutting-tomatoes-tips-from-the-kitchn-206686.

[127] Saurabh Bharti et al., "Preclinical Evidence for the Pharmacological Actions of Naringin: a Review," Planta medica (U.S. National Library of Medicine, April 2014), https://www.ncbi.nlm.nih.gov/pubmed/24710903.

88. TURMERIC

The Why:

Turmeric is a proven anti-inflammatory and pain-fighting herb that is helpful for people with rheumatoid arthritis.

Turmeric, the main spice in curry, is arguably the most powerful herb on the planet at fighting and potentially reversing disease. It has so many healing properties that currently there have been 6,235 peer-reviewed articles published proving the benefits of turmeric and one of its renowned healing compounds curcumin.

This puts turmeric on top of the list as one of the most frequently mentioned medicinal herbs in all of science.

The Science:

Turmeric has been used to treat diabetes in Ayurvedic and traditional Chinese Medicine for years. A 2013 review of scientific studies found that curcumin stabilizes glucose levels in the blood and also helped combat complications related to diabetes. In one study, 100 overweight people with type 2 diabetes took either 300 mg of curcumin or a placebo for 12 weeks. The researchers found that those taking curcumin had significantly lower fasting blood glucose.

There is promising research suggesting curcumin may reduce the risk of developing diabetes in high risk people too. In a 2012 study, all participants who took curcumin extract for nine months did not develop diabetes, although they were prediabetic. While 16% of the prediabetic participants who took a placebo did develop diabetes after the nine months.

The How:

You can grind the herb to add to soups, teas, and sauces.

The only problem with curcumin is that our liver inhibits most of its absorption, which decreases the effectiveness of the compound. The ways to increase the body's ability to absorb curcumin are as follows:

- Consume Turmeric with Beneficial Fats: Try consuming turmeric with healthy fats like avocado, olive oil, and coconut oil.
- Eat Turmeric with Quercetin: Quercetin is a plant flavonoid that inhibits the enzyme that deactivates curcumin.
- Mix Turmeric with Black Pepper: Curcumin absorption increases considerably more with just a small amount of piperine.[128,129]

[128] Nita Chainani-Wu, "Safety and Anti-Inflammatory Activity of Curcumin: a Component of Tumeric (Curcuma Longa)," Journal of alternative and complementary medicine (New York, N.Y.) (U.S. National Library of Medicine, February 2003), https://www.ncbi.nlm.nih.gov/pubmed/12676044.

[129] Dong-Wei Zhang et al., "Curcumin and Diabetes: a Systematic Review," Evidence-based complementary and alternative medicine : eCAM (Hindawi Publishing Corporation, 2013), https://www.ncbi.nlm.nih.gov/pmc/articles/PMC3857752/.

89. WATER

The Why:

Drinking enough water every day is good for overall health. Plain drinking water has zero calories and helps helps manage body weight and reduce caloric intake when substituted for drinks with calories, like regular soda. Drinking water can prevent dehydration, a condition that may cause unclear thinking, result in mood changes, your body to overheat, constipation, and kidney stones.

The Science:

A survey of 3,003 Americans found that 75 % likely suffered from chronic dehydration, due to net fluid loss. Although the survey found that Americans drank about eight servings of hydrating beverages per day, the hydration effects are offset by consumption of caffeinated beverages, alcohol, and a diet high in sodium.

A pair of recent studies found that young people who were mildly dehydrated were much more likely to feel fatigued during moderate exercise and even when sedentary. Unsurprisingly, fatigue is a common symptom of dehydration.

Even mild dehydration has been shown to put stress on our cognitive functioning. In young adults, for instance, dehydration was linked to a dip in concentration and short-term memory, as well as an increase in feelings of anxiety and irritability. With children, there are conclusive studies that show hydration improves attention and memory.

The How:

● Make that to-go.

When you're running tons of errands or juggling job responsibilities, it's harder to stay hydrated without giving in to convenience store or vending machine drink temptations. Fill a water bottle every morning and take it on your travels.

● Drink water before every meal or snack.

One simple way to increase water intake is to create this healthy habit: before each meal, even breakfast or a snack, drink a half glass or full glass of water. If you need a little flavor, add lemons, limes, or mint.

● Set a timer.

It sounds simple and maybe silly, but when the schedule is packed it's easy to forget to take care of yourself. Set reminders on your computer or smartphone to take regular water breaks.[130,131,132]

[130] Carol Kaesuk Yoon, "U.S. Drinking Itself Dry, Study Finds," The New York Times (The New York Times, June 16, 1998), https://www.nytimes.com/1998/06/16/science/us-drinking-itself-dry-study-finds.html.

[131] Matthew S. Ganio et al., "Mild Dehydration Impairs Cognitive Performance and Mood of Men," British Journal of Nutrition 106, no. 10 (July 2011): pp. 1535-1543, https://doi.org/10.1017/s0007114511002005.

[132] SkinnyMs., "12 Easy Ways to Increase Your Water Intake," Skinny Ms., April 13, 2019, http://skinnyms.com/12-easy-ways-to-increase-your-water-intake/.

90. WILD CAUGHT SALMON

The Why:

Wild Alaskan salmon is a powerhouse of nutrition. Consuming oily fish like wild Alaskan salmon once or twice a week may increase your lifespan by more than two years, and reduce your risk of dying from cardiovascular disease by 35%. This is because Alaskan salmon is a rich source of vitamins, minerals, lean protein and omega-3 fatty acids.

Just a 3-ounce serving of wild Alaskan salmon gives you 20% or more of the recommended daily allowance of vitamins B6 and B12, as well as niacin, which are all essential for metabolizing protein, carbohydrates and fats. These vitamins are needed to synthesize hormones and neurotransmitters, support nervous system function and regulate other nutrients in the body.

You can also get good amounts of selenium, magnesium and phosphorus from wild Alaskan salmon. Phosphorus and magnesium are both essential for bone health, while selenium helps inhibit free radical damage and ensure DNA and cellular tissue health.

Meanwhile, the omega-3 fatty acids in wild Alaskan salmon are said to be linked to a lower risk of high blood pressure, high blood cholesterol, heart arrhythmia and cardiovascular disease.

However, remember that to reap these benefits, you must make sure to get true wild Alaskan salmon, and not the inferior farmed salmon.

The Science:

Wild Alaskan salmon swim in the wild, where they can consume what nature intended for them to eat, resulting in a more complete nutritional profile. Meanwhile, farmed salmon are fed an unnatural diet of grain products and other ingredients, as explained by Science Line:

"Out in the ocean, salmon eat lots of small free-floating crustaceans, such as tiny shrimp. These crustaceans are filled with molecules called carotenoids, which show up as pigments all over the tree of life … It's these carotenoids that account for the reddish color of the salmon, as well as the pink color of flamingos and the red of a boiled lobster."

Farmed salmon, however, are not fed crustaceans. Instead, they eat dry pellets that look like dog food. According to the Atlantic Canada Fish Farmers Association, salmon chow includes ingredients such as 'soybean meal, corn gluten meal, canola meal, wheat gluten and poultry by-products.' Carotenoids, which are also essential for regular growth, can also be added to help give the fish its distinctive color.

These synthetic foods are not what Mother Nature intended for fish to consume, and changes the nutritional content of their flesh. Proof of this can be seen in the levels of omega-3 fats in farmed salmon, which are significantly lower – as much as 50% – than wild salmon.

In addition, farmed salmon have at least five times higher levels of omega-6 fat – throwingthe omega 3:6 ratio off-kilter, and wreaking havoc on people's health.

The How:

The Healthiest Way of Cooking Salmon
Salmon is best cooked with methods that will keep it moist and tender. It's easy to overcook and will become dry, so be sure to watch your cooking times.

One of our favorite ways to prepare salmon is our "Quick Broil" method.

Preheat the broiler on high and place an all stainless steel skillet (be sure the handle is also stainless steel) or cast iron pan under the heat for about 10 minutes to get it very hot.

Place salmon on hot pan and broil for 7-10 minutes, depending on thickness. You do not need to turn the salmon.

While grilled salmon tastes great, make sure it does not burn. It is best to grill salmon on a surface without a direct flame.

Extra care should be taken when grilling, as burning the fish damages nutrients and creates free radicals that may be harmful to your health.[133,134]

133 Michelle Bonham, "Marinated Wild Salmon Recipe," Allrecipes, May 17, 2007, https://www.allrecipes.com/recipe/84675/marinated-wild-salmon/.

134 Andrew Han, "Ever Wondered: Why Is Wild Salmon a Deeper Red than Farmed Salmon?," Scienceline, September 11, 2013, https://scienceline.org/2013/09/ever-wondered-why-is-wild-salmon-a-deeper-red-than-farmed-salmon/.

91. BIKE

The Why:

Take yourself on a bike ride. Bike riding is part of self-love and it is great exercise. It gets you into a new environment, increases your lung capacity, and lets you enjoy nature and yourself.

Cycling is mainly an aerobic activity, which means that your heart, blood vessels and lungs all get a workout. You will breathe deeper, perspire and experience increased body temperature, which will improve your overall fitness level.

The Science:

The health benefits of regular cycling include:

- Increased cardiovascular fitness.
- Increased muscle strength and flexibility.
- Improved joint mobility.
- Decreased stress levels.
- Improved posture and coordination.
- Strengthened bones.
- Decreased body fat levels.
- Prevention or management of disease.
- Reduced anxiety and depression.

The How:

Practice gliding down gentle slopes.

- Walk the bike to the top of a slope, mount it, and glide down, allowing the bike to slow naturally in the flat area at the bottom.
- Brake while gliding down hills.
- Try steering.
- Pedal through the bottom of the slope.
- Pedal up the slope. [135,136]

135 Person and wikiHow, "How to Ride a Bicycle," wikiHow (wikiHow, September 9, 2019), http://www.wikihow.com/Ride-a-Bicycle.

136 Department of Health & Human Services, "Cycling - Health Benefits," Better Health Channel (Department of Health & Human Services, November 30, 2013), https://www.betterhealth.vic.gov.au/health/healthyliving/cycling-health-benefits.

92. GROW A GARDEN

The Why:

Gardening in particular is associated with mental clarity and feelings of reward, and it has many physical benefits as well. Growing your own food can be particularly gratifying and an excellent source of fresh produce. From soil preparation to the joy of harvesting, there is always a task, big or small, during the growing season! If you have ever spent a summer gardening, you know that these tasks can serve as great exercise.

The Science:

A Dutch study asked two groups to complete a stressful task. Afterwards, one group gardened for 30 minutes, while the other group read indoors. Not only did the gardening group report better moods than the reading group, they also had measurably lower cortisol levels. Cortisol, "the stress hormone", may influence more than just mood: chronically elevated cortisol levels have been linked to everything from immune function to obesity, memory and learning problems, and heart disease. It may be more than brain hormones that cause higher self-esteem scores for gardeners: there's no more tangible measure of one's power to cause positive change in the world than to nurture a plant from seed to fruit-bearing.

The How:

• Plant in a sunny location. Vegetables need at least six hours of direct sunlight per day. The more sunlight they receive, the greater the harvest and the better the taste.

• Plant in good soil. Plants' roots penetrate soft soil easily, so you need nice loamy soil. Enriching your soil with compost provides needed nutrients. Proper drainage will ensure that water neither collects on top nor drains away too quickly.

• Space your crops properly. For example, corn needs a lot of space and can overshadow shorter vegetables. Plants set too close together compete for sunlight, water, and nutrition and fail to mature. Pay attention to the spacing guidance on seed packets and plant tabs.

• Buy high-quality seeds. Seed packets are less expensive than individual plants. If seeds don't germinate, your money—and time—are wasted. A few "extra" cents spent in spring for that year's seeds will pay off in higher yields at harvest time.[137]

[137] Agnes E. Van Den Berg and Mariëtte H.G. Custers, "Gardening Promotes Neuroendocrine and Affective Restoration from Stress - Agnes E. Van Den Berg, Mariëtte H.G. Custers, 2011," SAGE Journals, accessed October 1, 2019, http://journals.sagepub.com/doi/abs/10.1177/1359105310365577.

93. HIGH INTENSITY TRAINING

The Why:

Get your body to sweat, which removes toxins, burns stored glucose, and strengthens your heart. It's quick, can be fun, and you feel accomplished afterwards. You know it's a good workout when you can create a sweat angel.

The Science:

Most people aren't used to pushing into the anaerobic zone (that lovely place where you can't breathe and you feel like your heart is trying to jump out of your chest). But in this case, extreme training produces extreme results. One 2006 study found that after eight weeks of HIIT workouts, subjects could bicycle twice as long as they could before the study, while maintaining the same pace.

The How:

While there are no special rules for performing a HIIT routine, here are 5 Quick & Dirty Tips to get you started with your interval training:

1) Limit interval length to 2 minutes. If you're doing one of your hard intervals and you can go longer than 2 minutes, then you probably aren't exercising hard enough to generate a significant post-exercise calorie burning effect.

2) Go at least as long as 10 seconds. You can do efforts as short as 10 seconds, but remember: the shorter your intervals the more sets you'll need to do.

3) Beat boredom. You can mix things up during your HIIT routine. For example, do 3 hard efforts on the bike, then go over to the treadmill for 3 more, then move on to the elliptical trainer or rowing machines.

4) Combine with weight training. This can be as simple as doing jumping jacks and jumping as hard as you can for 30 seconds after each weight training set.

5) Recover. Remember, the purpose of HIIT is to allow you to go very hard during your intense intervals, and you won't be able to do that if you don't fully recover before each rep. I recommend at least a 1:2 interval to rest ratio, and up to a 1:4 interval to rest ratio. For example, a 1:2 interval to rest ratio would involve hard 60-second efforts following by easy 2 minute recovery periods.[138]

[138] Ben Greenfield, "How To Do High Intensity Interval Training," Quick and Dirty Tips (Get-Fit Guy, October 9, 2013), http://www.quickanddirtytips.com/health-fitness/exercise/how-to-do-high-intensity-interval-training?page=1.

94. GO ON A HIKE

The Why:

Hiking is for both exercise & self-love. It improves cardiorespiratory fitness (heart, lungs, blood vessels), muscular fitness, lowers risk of coronary heart disease & stroke, reduces depression and improves quality of sleep. Plus you get to be outdoors and in nature. The mental benefits of hiking will enhance the experience and have a tremendous benefit on your psyche when you return.

The Science:

According to a study published in Environmental Science & Technology, outdoor exercise is linked to "greater feelings of revitalization and positive engagement, decreases in tension, confusion, anger and depression, and increased energy."
For those with desk jobs and 40-hour weeks, getting outside provides a mental reset. You may set out to tone your glutes, but you're getting much more.

The How:
- Buy a local guidebook. Hiking guidebooks are essential when it comes to finding the right hike for you.
- Start small.
- Bring lots of water.
- Pack your backpack.
- Protect yourself from the sun.
- Wear the right shoes.
- Ask friends or family to join you.
- Know what to do in case of an emergency. [139,140]

[139] Alison Loughman, "Benefits of Hiking: There's Science behind the Feel-Good Workout," Boulder Daily Camera, August 5, 2014, http://www.dailycamera.com/get-out/ci_26280550/benefits-hiking-theres-science-behind-feel-good-workout.

[140] Thomas Churchill, "How to Hike," wikiHow (wikiHow, July 29, 2019), http://www.wikihow.com/Hike.

95. MARTIAL ARTS

The Why:

Martial arts are not just about getting stronger or losing weight; martial arts training can also help improve your mind. Here are some of the mental benefits associated with training in martial arts:

- Focus: Martial arts teach you to focus on your body and your actions, while tuning out distractions. This can translate directly into the rest of your life and allow you to stay more focused on the tasks at hand.

- Discipline: Martial arts teach you to control your emotions and impulses, and require great discipline and years of training to become proficient.

The Science:

In order to be a good martial artist, you must have very quick reflexes. Research has found that by participating in martial arts, you not only improve your reflexes while performing the activity, but actually experience faster reaction times during all activities of your life. This is very important in a number of daily activities, such as driving and even cooking.

The How:

Choosing a Discipline

While the benefits to martial arts training are numerous, so are the different disciplines and styles available. This can be overwhelming to those first entering the world of martial arts, but it doesn't have to be. Consider these questions when deciding on the right style for you:

What is your goal? What are you looking to get out of your training? Are you looking for the most effective way to defend against and deal damage? Then Krav Maga or a similar discipline may be for you. Are you looking to lose weight and get in shape? Cardiovascular focused kickboxing might be the right choice. Are you looking for competitive outlets? Try karate. Figure out what you want, determine your budget and find a discipline that fits these parameters.

96. OLYMPIC LIFTING

The Why:

Olympic-style weightlifting appears to be not just beneficial to athletes and weightlifters but also to the everyday exerciser. Whether you are trying to improve your sports performance, better your body composition, or just want a dynamic, full body workout, Olympic lifts are something that almost anyone can include in their exercise program.

Olympic-style weightlifting increases your power. Power is scientifically defined as the amount of force applied multiplied by the distance traveled divided by the time it takes. This is simply broken down as power being the ability to display strength with speed. The Olympic-style movements are great for enhancing this ability. Easy, simple, compound movements such as squats and deadlifts are important foundational exercises that help build a person's ability to promote power output. The power outputs of the Olympic lifts are significantly higher than those of basic exercises. So why do you need power? Powerful movements work the fast twitch fibers of the muscle, helping you to accelerate more quickly and recruit more muscle fibers to do work. Overall, having power makes you more efficient.

The Science:

Olympic lifting is one of the single best ways to improve jumping ability. In a study published in the Journal of Strength and Conditioning Research, subjects who performed Olympic lifts had higher counter movements jumps than subjects who performed power lifts. In fact, the Olympic group could jump higher than the power lifting group while jumping with 20 kilos (44 pounds) and 40 kilos (88 pounds) of additional load. Further, in an 8-week study JSCR (May 2005), this one comparing Olympic lifting to plyometric, the Olympic lifting

"…seemed to produce broader performance improvement than VJ (vertical jump) exercise in physically active subjects."[141]

The How:

Weightlifting is a lifestyle. It takes years of dedicated hours, reps, and methodical training to develop yourself into a stronger, more powerful, and technically-improved lifter. Every lifter has their own tips and advice that they could have used when they first started out. Taking the time to talk with more seasoned lifters and coaches will only help you throughout you weightlifting journey. Address your weaknesses, set strong foundations, and fight the urge to blindly sprint your way to your goals.

As coaches and athletes, we must all listen to our bodies. Programs are not created equal, and various variables exist within our training and recovery matrix. Closely monitoring day-to-day fluctuations, sleep patterns, nutritional status, bodyweight, long-term progress, and lifestyle stressors (work, family, etc) is important to fully customize your individual training program.

[141] Poliquin Group, "Top Five Benefits of Olympic Weightlifing," Poliquin Group, accessed October 1, 2019,
http://main.poliquingroup.com/Tips/tabid/130/EntryId/2295/Top-Five-Benefits-of-Olympic-Weightlifing.aspx.

97. QIGONG

The Why:

Qigong, a Chinese health practice based on gentle movements, meditation and breathing, has wide-ranging benefits, including improved balance, reduced blood pressure and even minimized depression symptoms.

The Science:

Initially many movements focus on gently opening and stretching the joints and muscles of the body, releasing tension that has often been there for years. By increasing the flow of blood and energy, the movement helps to fully nourish all parts of the body. Many of our students report that they feel very relaxed and energized after a session of QiGong, and that they sleep very deeply that night.

According to Chinese medicine, the energy relating to the body's internal organs flows around the extremities of the body - the hands and the feet. Thus by stretching the arms and legs in specific movements, the health of the internal organs can be improved.

The How:

The Qigong standing posture is one that you can work on at various times throughout the day. It is a relatively easy posture to practice and master and will build on other postures and promote confidence and overall well-being.

Stand upright with

- Your feet parallel and shoulder width distance.
- Knees slightly bent.
- Arms raised in front of your body with hands even to, or slightly below, your shoulders. - Elbows slightly bent.
- Hands foot lengths apart with palms pointed down. - Fingers separated and slightly curved. Pretend you are holding a ball in a relaxed manner.
- Eyes and mouth closed in a natural and unforced way.[142]

[142] WikiHow, "How to Practice Qigong," wikiHow (wikiHow, September 5, 2019), http://www.wikihow.com/Practice-Qigong.

98. SQUATTING

The Why:

Squats obviously help to build your leg muscles (including your quadriceps, hamstrings, and calves), but they also create an anabolic environment, which promotes body-wide muscle building.

In fact, when done properly, squats are so intense that they trigger the release of testosterone and human growth hormone in your body, which are vital for muscle growth and will also help to improve muscle mass when you train other areas of your body.

Squats actually help you improve both your upper and lower body strength.

The Science:
Based on a study the best way to perform a squat is to choose the most comfortable starting foot position, says Dr. Monica Rho, lead investigator and assistant professor at Northwestern University's Feinberg School of Medicine. "This will ensure that there's symmetrical loading of both legs during the squat."

The men and women in the study performed double-legged squats with their feet pointed forward at a fixed distance, in a mixed position with their feet at a fixed distance but in a self-selected position, and in a free position where subjects chose feet position and distance themselves.

As for how low you should go, Rho says, "There is a trade-off when it comes to deep squats. They tend to engage different muscles the deeper you go, however, the end knee and hip flexion can be detrimental to the joints over time."

Finally, Rho and her team observed whether squatting in front of a mirror helped the subject weight their legs equally. They found that with or without a mirror, healthy individuals don't tend to favor one leg during squats. The only time a mirror might help with loading, says Rho, is when you're recovering from a leg injury. People have a tendency to then favor their healthy leg, she adds, but that just leads to more injury.

The How:

Squats have long been criticized for being destructive to your knees, but research shows that when done properly, squats actually improve knee stability and strengthen connective tissue.

Warm up.

- Stand with your feet just over shoulder width apart.
- Keep your back in a neutral position, and knees centered over your feet.
- Slowly bend your knees, hips and ankles, lowering until you reach a 90-degree angle.
- Return to starting position -- repeat 15 to 20 times, for 2 to 3 sets for beginners (do this two or three times a week).
- Breathe in as you lower, breathe out as you return to starting position. [143,144]

[143] "How to Do Squats: 8 Reasons to Do Squat Exercises," Mercola.com, accessed October 1, 2019, http://fitness.mercola.com/sites/fitness/archive/2012/05/25/darin-steen-demonstrates-the-perfect-squat.aspx.

[144] Joel Seedman, "The Real Science of Squat Depth," T NATION, accessed October 1, 2019, https://www.t-nation.com/training/real-science-of-squat-depth.

99. GO FOR A WALK

The Why:

Take a walk! Simply taking a walk to break up your routine will begin to open up new ways of thinking, get some fresh oxygen in your lungs and your muscles moving. Walking isn't the end but the start of whatever new action you are looking to take.

The Science:

Walking helps you concentrate when your brain gets tired. The brain is basically a muscle with thoughts, and like other muscles it suffers from fatigue.

The stresses and strains of urban living, constant noise and dozens of things competing for our attention at any one time exacerbate what's been called "brain fatigue"- when you're distracted, absent-minded and have the attention span of a midge.

People have long understood intuitively that wandering through green space has a beneficial, calming impact on the mind, but a recent study in Scotland used technology to prove it. Lightweight brain-scanning devices were strapped to the heads of 12 people who were then sent on a walk through Edinburgh. The results showed that while busy, built-up areas induced frustration and irritation in the participants, green and parkland sections led to the brain becoming calmer and more meditative.

Naturally, this calmer state helps with brain fatigue. Jenny Roe, a lecturer at Heriot-Watt's School of the Built Environment, who oversaw the study, told the New York Times that while natural settings engage our brain, the type of engagement is effortless: "It's called involuntary attention in psychology. It holds our attention while at the same time allowing scope for reflection."

The How:

Start out warming up with a five-minute, slower paced walk. Start at a pace that's comfortable for you. Then gradually pick up speed until you're walking briskly — generally about 3 to 4 miles an hour. Slow your pace to cool down during the last five minutes of your walk.[145,146]

145 "Get Walking with This 12-Week Walking Schedule," Mayo Clinic (Mayo Foundation for Medical Education and Research, February 15, 2019), http://www.mayoclinic.org/healthy-lifestyle/fitness/in-depth/walking/art-20050972.

146 Harvard Health Publishing, "Walking: Your Steps to Health," Harvard Health, accessed October 1, 2019, http://www.health.harvard.edu/newsletter_article/Walking-Your-steps-to-health.

100. RESISTANCE TRAINING

The Why:

Resistance training (also called strength training or weight training) is the use of resistance to increase muscular contraction to build the strength, anaerobic endurance and size of skeletal muscles.

Resistance training is based on the principle that muscles of the body will work to overcome a resistance force when they are required to do so. When you practice resistance training repeatedly and consistently, your muscles become stronger.

A well-rounded fitness program includes strength training to improve joint function, bone density, muscle, tendon and ligament strength, aerobic exercise to improve your heart and lung fitness, and flexibility and balance exercises.

The Science:

There is impressive evidence in support of the theory that resistance training improves several major mental health issues. In addition, the research is convincing that resistance training can appreciably improve cognitive function. An exercise professional's bottom line message to clients is clear. For a mental lift, you should weight lift!

O'Connor, Herring and Caravalho (2010) summarize that the seven resistance training studies reviewed on this topic demonstrate that resistance training is a meaningful intervention for people suffering from anxiety. Interestingly, two of the seven studies compared the effects of high-intensity resistance training (exercises performed at 80% of 1-repetition maximum {1-RM}) versus moderate-intensity (50%-60% of 1-RM) and found that anxiety was better reduced with the moderate-intensity resistance training.

Mental Health Benefits from Resistance Training
Improved memory
Improved executive control
Reduced feelings of depression
Reduced chronic fatigue
Improved quality of sleep
Improved cognition
Decreased anxiety
Improved self-esteem

The How:

Strength Training

Lifting weights, using the weight machines at your health club, or doing calisthenics, are forms of strength or resistance training. You're working against some form of resistance. If using a set of "free" weights, your own body weight, or weight machines the goal is to stress a sequence of muscles and bones. According to the surgeon general, strength training at least twice a week is needed to stimulate bone growth.

Every gym has a trainer who can design a workout for your legs, back, shoulders, and arms and that's right for your fitness level. If you have any questions always seek to ask the professional. [147,148,149]

[147] Cay Anderson-Hanley, Joseph P. Nimon, and Sarah C. Westen, "Cognitive Health Benefits of Strengthening Exercise for Community-Dwelling Older Adults," Journal of Clinical and Experimental Neuropsychology 32, no. 9 (2010): pp. 996-1001, https://doi.org/10.1080/13803391003662702.

[148] Rebecca Buffum Taylor, "Weight-Bearing Exercise: 8 Workouts for Strong Bones," WebMD (WebMD), accessed October 1, 2019, http://www.webmd.com/osteoporosis/features/exercise-weight-bearing#3.

[149] Amenda Ramirez, "Resistance Training Improves Health," Resistance Training Improves Mental Health, 2010, https://www.unm.edu/~lkravitz/Article folder/RTandMentalHealth.html.

101. YOGA

The Why:

Yoga is part of a healthy life practice and for good reason. It will increase muscle strength and tone, and improve your respiration, energy and vitality. You don't need the latest yoga gear or a fancy studio to get started. All you have to do is choose to go and then do it.

The Science:

One NCCIH-funded study of 90 people with chronic low-back pain found that participants who practiced Iyengar yoga had significantly less disability, pain, and depression after six months.

In a 2011 study, also funded by NCCIH, researchers compared yoga with conventional stretching exercises or a self-care book in 228 adults with chronic low-back pain. The results showed that both yoga and stretching were more effective than a self-care book for improving function and reducing symptoms due to chronic low-back pain.

Conclusions from another 2011 study of 313 adults with chronic or recurring low-back pain suggested that 12 yoga classes every week resulted in better function than usual medical care.

The How:

Design a Home Yoga Practice

These six tips can help you chart a course for your home practice.

1. Start in a comfortable seated position. When you begin with stillness, you can see how your body and mind feel and then decide what you need today.

2. Pick a direction based on feeling, time allotment, intended outcome. If you're tired and pressed for time, choose a short restorative practice. If you're raring to go, opt for a more vigorous practice. If you need grounding and stability, focus on standing poses. If you need energy, incorporate backbends.

3. Set an intention. Ask, 'what do I want to get out of this time?" This simple suggestion ensures that you'll use your time—no matter how short—constructively. Sample intentions include creating a sense of spaciousness in a specific part of the body, working on a specific practice or pose, or noticing (and letting go of) any emotions that arise—without judgment.

4. Choose poses you love. If you want to build a consistent home practice, it has to be more of a carrot than a stick. Start by choosing four or five poses that feel great, so you'll feel compelled, rather than obligated, to roll out your mat.

5. Pay attention in class. Start taking mental notes in class: I really like when we do down dog, low lunge, down dog again, and pigeon, I'll do those three at home.

6. Move in all directions. Choose at least one pose for each direction the body moves—leaning side to side, forward and back, twisting, and turning upside down (which could be as simple as downward dog or a standing forward bend). If you incorporate all the directions, you create a complete practice.[150,151]

[150] "Yoga for Beginners," Yoga Journal, April 3, 2017, http://www.yogajournal.com/category/beginners/.

[151] Kate Hanley, "The Beginner's Guide to Home Yoga Practice," Yoga International (Yoga International, May 21, 2013), https://yogainternational.com/article/view/the-beginners-guide-to-home-yoga-practice.